SIMPLE STEPS

The Chinese Way to Better Health

Lynn Jaffee, L.Ac.

ISBN: 1-4392-1836-6

ISBN-13: 9781439218365

Visit www.booksurge.com to order additional copies.

TABLE OF CONTENTS

ACKNOWLEDGEMENTS

I wish to thank the following people without whose help this book would never have come into being: Stephanie Ross, for pushing me to write; Judy Mahle Lutter and Randy Victor for their generous editing skills; Shelley Conn, my practice partner, for her patience and insight; all of my teachers of Chinese medicine; and Steve, Michael, and Andrew for their support and love.

INTRODUCTION

Several summers ago, I happened to pick up a back issue of *People* magazine. One article featured a picture of actress Gwyneth Paltrow in an evening gown at an award gala. Besides the gown, she was sporting dark circles on her back from a Chinese treatment called cupping, which is painless but leaves a mark. The point of the article was that Paltrow had discovered Chinese medicine and had the marks to prove it. Since then, it seems that articles in the popular press appear almost weekly describing some celebrity or athlete who has been helped by acupuncture. In 2007 Oprah had an acupuncturist demonstrate the wonders of this ancient healing art on her show. Dr. Andrew Weil, the Mayo Clinic, the World Health Organization, and many other prominent individuals and institutions have hailed the use of acupuncture as a safe, natural and effective method of healing.

The reality is that an increasing number of health consumers are turning to Chinese medicine for some aspect of their health care. Many want to understand how this medicine works and how they can incorporate it into their daily lives. This is no easy task, primarily because it involves a very different and foreign...well, Chinese...way of looking at health, and at the world in general. In addition, Chinese medicine is composed of several modalities, and each one has its own theories and methods of practice.

In my acupuncture practice, I find myself explaining the concepts of Chinese medicine to patients on a daily basis. Most are fascinated and many want more information. I have found that the pamphlets in my waiting room that give a brief overview of this medicine are too simple for many of my patients, and books that I have recommended offer too much information, require more of a commitment in reading time, and can be confusing and overwhelming.

I first tried acupuncture when a nagging muscle pull had not responded to Western biomedical treatment. I remember looking at the wall charts in my practitioner's office depicting the Five Elements and the energetic pathways of the body and thinking about how mysterious Chinese medicine seemed. One goal in writing this book is to take some of the mystery out of Chinese medicine and create an introduction to the basic theories on which it is based.

The Chinese sages have written that when you experience health problems, you should first try to solve them through diet and lifestyle changes. If those changes don't resolve the problem, then you should turn to acupuncture and Chinese herbs for help. In that spirit, I have included some self-assessment tools that will guide you in understanding your own body patterns, along with some simple lifestyle actions that may be helpful in achieving mind/body balance and improving your health.

This book is not intended to diagnose a medical condition, nor is it meant to be used as a substitute for working with an experienced practitioner of Chinese medicine. If you have a health concern, you should seek the care of a Western physician.

In some instances I have included case studies to illustrate a point. The names and identifying details in each case have been changed to protect those individuals.

This book is meant to be a primer and a workbook using the theories of Chinese medicine. I hope that you will use the ideas presented here to create a more meaningful dialogue with your own acupuncturist or TCM practitioner as well as to bring your awareness of the patterns and cycles of your body to a new level.

CHAPTER 1

WHAT IS CHINESE MEDICINE?

Simply stated, Chinese medicine is a system of healing that originated in China thousands of years ago, and is still used in many parts of the world today. Most people think Chinese medicine is acupuncture—and they are right, up to a point. Chinese medicine actually encompasses several modalities, or systems of healing, including herbal medicine, a kind of bodywork called *Tui Na*, dietary therapy, lifestyle habits, a system of movement called *Qi Gong*, and *Feng Shui*—the energetics of the environment. However, the part of Chinese medicine that we are most familiar with in the United States is acupuncture.

CHINESE AND WESTERN MEDICINE: A COMPARISON

One of the first things I learned as I began studying Chinese medicine was that I should not try to think of Chinese medicine in Western terms, and for good reason. Both systems of healing have their benefits and drawbacks, but they are otherwise nothing alike.

Western medicine is based on scientific study, and is generally best for the treatment of acute conditions, using drugs or surgery as the first line of defense against disease. Western medicine treats symptoms very well, but in many cases does not cure the illness. If the symptoms of an illness go away after a Western treatment, it tends to be a temporary fix, or other symptoms will arise at some future point. For example, the use of antidepressant medications has increased dramatically over the past several decades and can be effective in reducing the symptoms of depression. However, the patients I have seen in my clinic who take these drugs generally do not like the side effects and want to stop taking these medications. Unfortunately, they find that their depression returns when they decrease their dosage or stop taking the medication altogether. For them, it seems to be a tradeoff between being depressed or having unwanted drug side effects. To me, this is not a cure.

Chinese medicine is based on observation, and tends to be a better choice in treating some chronic illnesses, using a variety of modalities. It treats the underlying cause of an illness, and in doing so also treats the symptoms. In addition, Chinese medicine treats the whole person, taking into account not only the physical aspects of a patient, but also the emotional and spiritual.

It is important to note that organ systems, such as the Spleen or Heart; vital substances such as Qi or Blood; and elements such as Earth or Wood are capitalized in Chinese medicine. This is because these terms refer to more than just body parts or elements in nature. These terms are essential systems in Chinese medicine and are capitalized in acknowledgement of their importance. In contrast, the spleen, heart, blood, and the elements in a Western context are not capitalized. In addition, the term "elements" in a Western scientific context refer to chemical substances reduced to their simplest essences. However, in Chinese medicine, the elements are phases in nature that describe relationships and qualities within the body.

Treatments in the Western medical model usually work very quickly, but either tend to have side effects from prescription drugs or problems resulting from surgery. In contrast, Chinese medical treatments tend not to have any side effects and are generally considered safe. The downside of Chinese medicine is that because it balances the body to promote self-healing, it can take time to be effective.

The bottom line is that there is a time and a place for both Chinese and Western medicine. In addition, the two systems are not mutually exclusive. They can work as complementary systems of healing, which means that they can work well together, depending on the circumstances. Sometimes Western medicine may be a better choice for care, and at other times Chinese medicine will be more appropriate or effective.

THE SYMBOLIC NATURE
OF CHINESE MEDICINE

The foundations of Chinese medicine are based on our relationship with nature. A basic concept of this medicine is that we are miniature models of the earth and the universe, and as such exhibit some of the same characteristics as the natural world around us. In fact, much of the language of Chinese medicine parallels the weather, seasons, and other natural phenomena. Illnesses can be described as warm, cold, damp, wind, dryness and even summerheat. The body's organs correspond to natural elements such as Earth, Fire, Wood, Water, and Metal. As a result, much of what is understood about the body is described in metaphor.

When we talk about organs in a Western medical context, we are talking about a specific physical organ. It has a shape and is located in pretty much the same place in everyone, and if you were on the operating table, we could actually remove it. When we talk about specific organs in the context of the Chinese medical model, we are describing symbolic systems of functioning. For example, the Spleen is an organ that governs digestion. However, the function of the Spleen is much broader than simply digesting food. It is an organ system that takes food in, separates food from liquids, turns food into energy and blood, metabolizes liquids, nourishes your flesh (muscles), and holds things in place. So a person with a weak Spleen system might experience digestion problems. However, problems might also be experienced that are seemingly unrelated to digestion, such as low energy, water retention, poor muscle tone, and easy bruising—all part of a *pattern* related to the function of the Spleen.

This is a really important idea to keep in mind. In later sections, as you read about the organs, try to keep Chinese and Western medicine separate, keep your thinking flexible, and try not to compare the Chinese Spleen to the one your doctor can remove if you rupture it in a sledding accident.

PATTERNS OF IMBALANCE

If you visit a practitioner of Chinese medicine for a specific symptom, you might be surprised to be asked all kinds of questions that seem to have absolutely nothing to do with your symptom. In fact, you may become impatient as your practitioner asks you about your bowel movements when you are there to be treated for acne. However, for your practitioner to arrive at an accurate diagnosis, he or she must have a complete picture of your internal makeup. Your symptom is simply a manifestation of an imbalance, and to treat it correctly your practitioner will put that symptom into the context of a pattern in order to treat the source of the imbalance.

It is interesting that a single symptom can be a manifestation of very different patterns in different people. For example, three people may come to my office wanting to be treated for insomnia. The first, a busy executive, explains that he has difficulty falling asleep because his mind is racing when he goes to bed. He shares that he frequently feels stressed by his job, and when he gets home, he's irritable with his family. He says he feels thirsty, and his face appears red. This man would be diagnosed with a pattern called a stagnation of Liver energy, which is causing heat and restlessness.

The second person to be treated for insomnia is a smallish woman who is about fifty years old. She reports that while she can fall asleep at night, she wakes about 3:00 a.m. with night sweats and has difficulty getting back to sleep. She also complains that she has a chronic dull ache in her lower back and that her knees feel weak. Her face is pale, but her cheeks are red. This woman's insomnia is due to a pattern of depleted Kidney Yin.

The third person with insomnia is a woman in her thirties, who had surgery about six months ago for appendicitis. She complains that her sleep is restless all night long, and she wakes frequently. She also has heart palpitations, occasional dizziness, dry skin and brittle nails. Her face looks pale and drawn. This woman's sleep problem is caused by a depletion of Blood.

All three of these people would be diagnosed with insomnia in Western biomedicine, and would most likely be prescribed a sleep aid. However, in the Chinese medical model, the only thing these three people have in common is that their imbalance is manifesting as insomnia. For each, the underlying cause of their insomnia is different from the others, and each would be treated with acupuncture and herbal prescriptions unique to the particular imbalance.

WHAT CAN CHINESE MEDICINE TREAT?

For about two thousand years, Chinese medicine was the *only* system of healing in China. It was used not only for pain relief, but also as internal medicine, treating everything from digestive problems to anxiety. Western medicine's influence in China is only decades old.

Today, more and more Western medical institutions are recognizing the effectiveness of acupuncture and Chinese herbs for a limitless number of conditions. The World Health Organization has listed dozens of conditions that acupuncture can treat effectively.

Many hospitals in the United States are adding acupuncture to their list of services. Acupuncture has been featured in all levels of the media from the *Mayo Clinic Women's Healthsource*, to the *Today Show*, to Dr. Andrew Weil's books.

CHAPTER 2
MODALITIES OF CHINESE MEDICINE

A BRIEF HISTORY

Traditional Chinese medicine has a very long, rich history that has survived and thrived for thousands of years. While this medicine continues to evolve, many of the concepts that were in practice centuries ago are still in use today.

Historians believe that Chinese medicine began as a way to treat conditions in the body involving heat, such as fever or infections. It's believed that early practitioners used sharpened stones to drain infections or to bleed points on the body to reduce fevers. Some of the most important texts on Chinese medicine written centuries ago describe the stages of febrile disease (illnesses involving a fever) with very specific ways to treat each stage of illness. These texts give us insight into the earliest uses of Chinese medicine, as well as theories that are the foundation of acupuncture as it is practiced today.

The original stone points became obsolete with the discovery of metallurgy. When early practitioners began using metal, the points became finer and sharper, ultimately evolving into the acupuncture needles that we use today. While acupuncture was practiced throughout China, other modalities developed regionally. In the north of China, where the weather is cold and dry, the use of moxabustion was developed. Moxabustion is a method of warming parts of your body, usually acupuncture points, with burning herbs. It was used for illnesses that were considered cold in nature, such as joint pain and other conditions which are aggravated by cold weather. Today moxabustion is still used in acupuncture clinics by burning the herb artemesia near specific points of the body to achieve a warming effect. Sadly, many acupuncturists must use other warming methods, because moxabustion smells strongly like marijuana and is very penetrating, which poses a problem in most modern office buildings.

With its warmer climate, southern China was the origin of a different kind of healing method. The temperate climate and fertile soil in the South are ideal for thousands of varieties of trees and plants to flourish. As a result, herbal medicine developed in the South, and over the centuries spread throughout China. Today Chinese herbal medicine is an important and commonly used treatment method.

Much of what we know about Chinese medicine today comes from ancient texts that were written by practitioners of acupuncture or herbalists hundreds and sometimes thousands of years ago. It is interesting to note that the ancients did not perform dissection in order to understand the human body. Instead, they observed the body and relationships between various bodily functions, the seasons, foods, emotions and the universe in general. Over the centuries, the body of knowledge that comprises Chinese medicine continued to grow as royal physicians and rural practitioners alike shared successful methods of treatment.

Even today Chinese medicine continues to evolve as practitioners share their clinical successes. However, unlike Western medicine, in which a new theory is often thought to disprove what was previously known, new ideas in Chinese medicine are simply considered a new layer of understanding. As a result, Chinese medicine is constantly evolving, but the ancient ideas upon which the medicine was built are still considered the foundation. They are to be studied and revered as such.

ACUPUNCTURE

One of the cornerstones of Chinese medicine is the practice of acupuncture, which is the insertion of fine needles into points on your body to stimulate self-healing. Acupuncture works by manipulating your body's energy, which makes it hard for some people to accept. However, you may remember from seventh grade biology that the mitochondria in our cells manufacture energy. We know that energy is a power even at the molecular level. The Chinese simply believe that some of this energy moves in pathways in your body. Pain, illness, or uncomfortable symptoms arise when this energy is either blocked or depleted.

An example of blocked energy is when someone is having a heart attack. In many cases, a common symptom of a heart attack, especially for men, is pain in the left arm. While the blockage is in the heart, the pain that is radiating down the arm is in what is known in Chinese medicine as the Heart pathway. Another example of blocked energy is the stiff neck and shoulders that many people experience when they are stressed out. The stress causes tightness which inhibits the flow of blood and energy, creating the pain and stiffness, which can also travel elsewhere and cause headaches or chronic back pain.

The effects of depleted energy on your body may look a bit like low energy in Western medicine. Fatigue or poor energy levels tend to be hallmark symptoms in either system of medicine. However, in Chinese medicine, depleted energy also means that your body doesn't have the energy to carry out internal functions, like digestion or the ability to breathe efficiently. As a result, symptoms of depleted energy may also include digestive problems or shortness of breath.

This energy moving throughout your body pools or rises to the surface at various points, called acupoints. An acupuncturist can access this energy by inserting needles into various acupoints to either unblock energy or help build up depleted energy.

In addition, while the pathways rise to the surface of your body, they also run deep to your internal organs. As a result, an acupuncturist can access your internal organs through the acupoints on your body's surface.

It's important to be clear that your acupuncturist is not using needles as "medicine." Rather, by inserting needles into appropriate points, your acupuncturist is stimulating your body to heal itself. Think of your acupuncturist as a facilitator, but remember, you are doing the work of healing.

There are many different styles of acupuncture beyond the traditional Chinese style. As the practice of acupuncture moved outside of China, other styles developed in several Asian countries. As a result, Japanese style acupuncture, Korean Hand acupuncture, and Vietnamese acupuncture are all in practice today. There are also several schools of thought that have evolved from traditional Chinese acupuncture, such as five-phase style and auricular (ear) acupuncture. All of these styles use thin needles to balance your body's energy.

CHINESE HERBAL MEDICINE

Another cornerstone of Chinese medicine is the use of herbs. Almost as old as acupuncture, Chinese herbal medicine is an effective healing modality in its own right.

The theory behind herbal medicine is that each herb exerts several different effects on the body. Each herb has an inherent temperature, action, and organ(s) that it affects. For example, ginger is a warming herb that helps resolve colds and flu, calms the stomach, stops vomiting, and helps to warm the lungs and stop coughing.

Generally, herbs are combined in formulas to achieve specific actions. Herbs are combined because usually no one herb has all the desired actions. Several herbs may be chosen and combined into a formula to augment or offset each other's actions. For example, two herbs with similar actions might be combined for maximum effect, or if a very warm herb is used in a formula, a smaller amount of a slightly cooling herb might be included to offset the warming effect of the first. By combining herbs in this way, practitioners can ensure that side effects are minimal.

Traditionally, herbs were combined with water and boiled to make a decoction (tea). In more recent times, the decoction might be dried and formed into a powder, or boiled down and formed into pills. Herbal medicine is a great way to augment or extend the effects of an acupuncture treatment. In addition, as a patient's condition changes, the herbal formula can be fine-tuned by adding, deleting, or changing the amounts of herbs in the formula.

DIETARY THERAPY

Like herbs, foods have inherent properties. They can have an effect on a particular organ and can have an inherent temperature, meaning they can cool or warm your body. For example, a practitioner might prescribe watermelon, cucumbers, or tomatoes for their cooling properties. In fact, there is an overlap between herbal medicine and dietary therapies. There are a number of foods that are used in herbal formulas, including scallions, walnuts, sesame seeds, certain melons, and sea vegetables. While there are some similarities between herbs and foods, most foods, including those mentioned above, tend to have weaker effects than those of herbs. This is because herbal formulas are more concentrated, while foods are eaten in larger quantities and more frequently.

Food is considered a kind of medicine that you eat three times a day, and illness can occur if you do not eat the right foods; if you eat too much or too little; or if your foods are not cooked properly. Dietary therapy is often the first line of defense in Chinese medicine. In theory, practitioners should treat their patients first through food therapy and lifestyle changes. If patients do not get better, then they should be treated with herbs and acupuncture. In reality, however, dietary therapy is frequently combined with acupuncture and herbal medicine for the best results.

CUPPING

The purpose of cupping is to move energy and facilitate healing. It involves placing glass or plastic cups on the body in which some kind of vacuum has been created. The vacuum acts to pull the skin, increasing the flow of blood and energy. For practical reasons, cupping is usually done on larger areas of the body such as your back or legs; but it can be done almost anywhere on the body, if necessary.

There are a couple of ways to create a vacuum in the cups. One is by using cups with small gaskets through which air can be pulled out with a pump. The other method is called fire cupping. A cotton ball is soaked in alcohol and lit, then held in the cup for a few seconds until the flame has used up all the air. Then the cup is quickly placed on the skin. It sounds very dramatic and dangerous, but it is actually quite safe and works very well. The cups may then be left on the skin for five to ten minutes, or they can be moved across the skin (retaining the vacuum) to treat a larger area.

The downside of cupping is that the cups leave a mark on the skin that looks like a perfectly round bruise. If you are planning to wear strapless evening wear, you may want to postpone being cupped until your next visit.

BODYWORK, MOVEMENT, AND THE WORLD AROUND YOU

Another frequently used modality of Chinese medicine is a kind of bodywork called *Tui Na*. While it may feel a bit like a massage to the recipient, practitioners of Tui Na use several kinds of hand movements, strokes, and pushing along your energetic points and pathways to move energy and promote healing. Tui Na may be used for a variety of conditions, but it is primarily a technique for addressing musculoskeletal pain.

Many practitioners of Chinese medicine will incorporate the practice of *Qi Gong* into their treatment plans. Translated as "energy cultivation," Qi Gong is an intricate series of movements that looks much like *Tai Qi*. The movements are designed to strengthen particular organs, cultivate Qi (energy), stimulate energy pathways, and strengthen the body. Like Yoga or any of the martial arts, Qi Gong is meant to be practiced daily.

In the Chinese tradition, the world around you also has an impact on energy and how you feel. The practice of geomancy, or *Feng Shui*, involves assessing your surroundings and making specific changes to energetically enhance your space. For example, if you walk into a friend's house that is cluttered, you may feel scattered and uncomfortable. However, if you walk into a house with few distractions and simple furnishings, it will give you an entirely different feeling.

The art of Feng Shui is about changing your space, whether your home, yard, office, or the like, to best suit your purposes. You may want to enhance your home to promote marital harmony and security. In contrast, you may want to change the layout of your office to encourage prosperity or to "open the door" to more clients.

While the modalities of Chinese medicine may feel strange and foreign, I encourage you to open your mind to the possibility of thinking differently about your world. These systems have been in use for thousands of years, and they still exist because of their effectiveness and acceptance in many parts of the world.

CHAPTER 3
UNDERSTANDING QI AND BLOOD

Qi (pronounced chee) is one of the fundamental forces in your body and in the universe, according to Chinese theory. The concept of Qi is difficult to translate, and many compare it to the term "energy." However, Qi is much more than energy.

In the broadest sense, Qi is the motivational force that affects everything in the universe. It's the force that guides the planets in our solar system and the movement of atoms on a microscopic level. Everything has Qi, including inanimate objects. It is also the driving energy behind any change or transformation. For example, the life cycle of a tree is governed by Qi, which is responsible for its growth, seasonal changes, and decomposition at the end of its life.

In addition, Qi animates matter. In this context, Qi might be considered the life force of all living things. As an extension of this concept, Qi takes on a number of qualities in your body:

- Qi is transformative. This means that Qi is necessary for such processes as digestion to take place. Essentially, Qi is the magic ingredient by which the foods you eat and fluids you drink become nutrients and living tissue.

- Qi is warming. Your body exists at a very narrow temperature range of about 98 degrees, give or take about five degrees. The action of Qi provides that warmth.

- Qi is moving. This means that any activity within your body, such as the movement of internal organs (digestion and peristalsis, for example) and the movement of muscles and tendons, is powered by Qi. Your body in motion is also powered by Qi.

- Qi is protective. Much like the immune system, Qi protects you from outside pathogens which cause colds and the flu.

- Qi holds things. In your body, your organs are held up, blood is held in the vessels, babies are held in the uterus, and food is held in your digestive tract. All of these processes are provided by Qi.

WHAT DOES QI HAVE TO DO WITH MY HEALTH?

The short answer is that when you are healthy, plentiful Qi moves throughout your body in the pathways and organs without obstruction. When you become ill or have pain or uncomfortable symptoms, Qi is usually involved. Either Qi isn't moving freely, or there's not enough Qi to power the everyday functions of your body.

To assess how well Qi is doing its job in your body, put a check beside each of the following statements that is true for you.

Section 1

____I frequently experience joint or muscle pain.

____I tend to feel frustrated.

____My life is pretty stressful.

____I get lots of tension headaches.

____(Women) I have painful menstrual periods.

____I often feel sad or depressed.

____I feel pain around my ribs.

____I struggle with the way my life is and how I want it to be.

____I feel like I have a lump in my throat.

____I get angry frequently, or people tell me I have a "short fuse."

____I sigh a lot.

____I have a hard time sleeping because my mind is racing.

Total for Section 1_____

Section 2

____I get sick frequently.

____After I eat, I feel tired.

____I tend to bruise easily.

____I feel colder than most other people.

____My appetite is not very good.

____My voice is soft.

____I am frequently tired.

____My energy fluctuates broadly over the course of the day.

____I get out of breath when I'm barely exerting myself.

____I feel gassy and bloated after I eat.

____I sweat during the day, even though I'm not exercising.

____I have a pale or sallow complexion.

Total for Section 2_____

Total your score for each of the above sections. If you have more than two or three items checked in a section, or if you checked a lot of items in one section and few or none in the other, then the following discussion is appropriate for you.

Section 1

All of the items in this section are indications of an energy blockage somewhere in your body. The most common symptom of energy, or Qi, not moving freely is pain. Whether you are having muscle or joint pain, headaches, or painful menstrual cramps, your body is giving you a heads-up that your energy is blocked.

The movement of Qi throughout your body should be smooth and seamless. However, when Qi becomes blocked, your emotions usually are playing a role. Very strong and uncontrolled emotions can cause Qi to stagnate.

A number of questions in Section I deal with Qi stagnation related to your emotions. Emotional blockage is a kind of Qi constraint, in which there is a difference between how you want things to be and how they actually are. It is important to understand that an emotional Qi blockage will ultimately manifest itself physically. People who are unhappy with their lives, stressed, depressed or anxious create an imbalance that will lead to physical symptoms, such as digestive problems, insomnia, pain or headaches, to name a few.

On the flip side, physical stagnation can build up emotional pressure that may manifest as strong and uncontrollable emotions. For example, some women experience Qi stagnation around the time of their menstrual cycle—a time when hormones, blood and energy should move smoothly. If Qi is not moving freely during this time, the results are emotional symptoms such as PMS with irritability, sadness, or anger. Stagnation can also generate physical symptoms such as menstrual cramps, back pain and breast tenderness.

Several years ago, Maria came into my clinic for treatment because she was feeling stressed and irritable, and was having trouble getting to sleep at night. Maria was a pretty, well-dressed woman in her late thirties. She worked as a project manager at a large advertising company. During the course of her first visit, she revealed that she was unhappy at her job, but was unwilling to leave because it paid well. She also described how she was unhappy with her short fuse. She did not like that she was impatient at home with her husband and children. She described herself as a very busy person with a lot to do, both at work and at home.

I asked Maria about her energy levels, and she described having the sensation of too much energy. When she got into bed at night, Maria said, her mind would race, making it hard for her to calm down enough to be able to fall asleep.

Eventually she would drop off and stay asleep for the rest of the night. Maria's symptoms were somewhat better when she exercised regularly, and were always worse during the week before her period.

I diagnosed Maria with a pattern of Qi stagnation. I treated her with acupuncture, and after the first treatment, she reported feeling less "wound up." I also prescribed an herbal formula for Maria and some simple methods to relieve stress. After three treatments, Maria reported back to me that she was getting to sleep easily at night, and her family noticed that she was a lot less irritable.

WHAT YOU CAN DO

If you have blocked Qi, acupuncture can be one of the most effective remedies. However, there are some things that you can do on your own to help your energy move more freely. In general, movement of some kind is helpful in unblocking stagnant Qi, and moving your body falls into this category. All kinds of movement or exercise are effective, whether it is aerobic exercise such as running or playing tennis or something more calming, such as stretching or Tai Qi. Even taking a walk is helpful.

When Qi stagnation takes the form of sore or tight muscles, massage can be an effective way to get things moving. Massage opens your pathways and helps to improve circulation of both Qi and Blood, and it feels good. In most cases, the effects of massage are temporary, but the relief it brings is very real.

If the source of your stagnation is emotional in nature, then quiet breathing exercises, meditation, visualization, or any other regular stress-busting activity will help unblock your energy. The key here is finding an enjoyable routine that you can maintain on a regular basis. In addition, working to change a situation which is causing strong emotions—either by changing an untenable situation or by changing your reaction to the situation—is a way of addressing the stagnation at its core.

31

Some people drink coffee as a way to get things moving. Coffee actually works to move energy in the short term, but drinking too much of it can ultimately deplete your energy and leave you feeling sluggish when the caffeine has worn off.

Many of my patients say they feel better when they get into a regular routine of physical activity paired with some kind of quiet, meditative time to themselves. Whether your body craves exercise, quiet time, or certain foods, it will tell you what it needs; you just have to listen.

Section 2

If you checked several of the items in Section 2, chances are pretty good that your Qi is depleted. One of the most frequent signs of depleted Qi is the most obvious—low energy. Feeling fatigued, experiencing energy fluctuations over the course of the day, feeling tired after eating a meal, getting out of breath easily, and a weak voice are all indications that your Qi is low.

Another function of Qi is to protect your body from outside elements, such as colds and flu. So if you feel like you are sick all the time, chances are that the protective aspect of your Qi is not up to par. A further protective function of Qi is to regulate the opening and closing of your pores. Some people with weak Qi will sweat during the course of the day with very little exertion, even if they feel cold (remember, Qi is warming).

A few items in Section 2 deal with appetite and digestion. One of the functions of your Spleen organ system is to digest food and liquids and convert them into energy (Qi) and nutrients. If you have depleted Qi, chances are that your Spleen organ system either is not getting the right foods or is not efficiently converting the food you eat into energy. This is another case in which one imbalance can cause the other and vice versa. If your Spleen is not digesting well, then you aren't making adequate Qi. However, if your Qi is depleted, your digestive system will suffer. Loss of appetite, gas and bloating, heartburn, and loose stools are all indicators of weak Spleen Qi. See Chapter 6 for more on the Spleen.

Bruising easily is a common manifestation that the holding function of Qi is deficient, because it is not containing your blood within the vessels. In addition, feeling cold or exhibiting a pale, sallow complexion can be indications that Qi isn't warming your body adequately.

What causes your energy to become depleted? Many things! In fact, just about anything that tires you out, stresses your body or wears on your mind can deplete your Qi. Examples include working or studying too hard, too much exercise, or a stressful job or home life. Also, your Qi can get depleted if you aren't building it up properly. The best ways to build Qi are through diet, digestion, and feeding yourself spiritually and mentally.

Maureen was a thirty-four-year-old woman who came to my office seeking treatment for chronic fatigue syndrome, from which she had been suffering for over twelve years.

Maureen explained that she was so tired in the morning that it became impossible for her to hold a job unless it began later in the day. She was becoming quite worried because it was difficult to find and keep a job that would accommodate her schedule. Over several years, Maureen had tried all kinds of remedies and supplements to boost her energy, to no avail. As we spoke, I noticed that Maureen's face appeared pale, she spoke with a weak voice, and she said she always felt cold.

Maureen was usually too exhausted to cook nutritious meals for herself, and her diet consisted of fast foods and sandwiches, with few fruits and vegetables. She had very little appetite, her digestion was poor, and her energy dropped after eating a meal.

I treated Maureen for several months for a deficiency of Qi. Along with acupuncture, I made some lifestyle and dietary suggestions that would improve Maureen's energy. Over time, she regained some of her energy, but because her diet never changed, the improvements were not long-lasting, and Maureen continued to struggle with her symptoms.

WHAT YOU CAN DO

If your Qi is depleted, the key is to protect the Qi you have while trying to rebuild more through lifestyle and diet. Qi is made from the food you eat and the air you breathe, so diet, digestion, breathing, and good posture all play a role in rebuilding depleted Qi.

Digestion is every bit as important to your health as what you eat. If you have digestive problems, try to choose whole grains, fruits, and vegetables with small amounts of protein instead of fast, pre-prepared or packaged foods. In addition, you will better digest foods that are cooked, such as soups, stews, and stir-fried dishes. Your body uses more energy warming and digesting cold or raw foods, so until your digestion is back on track, try to limit those foods as much as possible.

According to Daverick Leggett (*Recipes for Self-Healing*; see "Learning More"), specific foods that enhance Qi tend to be slightly sweet and warm in nature. Root vegetables, such as yams and sweet potatoes, along with pumpkins and squash, legumes (beans), some nuts and seeds, and most vegetables are Qi-enhancing. In general, locally grown, organic foods and produce in season tend to have more nutrients, and to be more energy building, than chemically treated foods. Qi- promoting herbs should be prescribed by an experienced herbalist on a case-by-case basis, because each person will have different organ imbalances, but sage and thyme used in meal preparation are appropriate for most people.

Most of us do not think much about breathing because it's something we do all the time. However, knowing that in part Qi is made from the air you take into your body through the lungs might make you a little more conscious of how you breathe. Take a few minutes each day to take a deep breath, open your chest as you breathe in, hold for five seconds or so, and release slowly until your lungs are empty. Repeat this sequence for five breaths. During the course of the day, check your posture—you can't breathe properly (or digest well) if you are slumped over a keyboard or folded into a couch.

Rest and rejuvenation are also important components of rebuilding depleted Qi. Make sure you take time each day to feed yourself mentally and spiritually. This may be as simple as taking some time to walk outside, read a book, or play an instrument. Equally important is getting enough sleep—eight hours a night is ideal. If you struggle with insomnia, consulting with a practitioner of Chinese medicine can be extremely helpful.

IF YOU CHECKED SEVERAL ITEMS IN BOTH SECTIONS

If you checked a number of items in both Section 1 and Section 2, then it is likely that stagnation is depleting your Qi. This is a frequent pattern when people are stressed, emotionally upset, or in a lot of pain.

Key Terms

Stagnation is a blockage in your body. Necessary substances like Qi, Blood, Yin, or Yang can become blocked. However, pathogens such as phlegm or heat can also stagnate. A stagnation or blockage is considered a pattern of excess which needs to be moved, cleared, or resolved.

Pathogens are the cause of disease in Chinese medicine. They act like bad weather in your body, causing imbalances that trigger symptoms and illnesses. Viruses and bacteria can also act as pathogens.

Depletion or deficiency occurs when one or more of the necessary substances in your body are in short supply. In this case, the appropriate action is to tonify, nourish, or build up the depleted substance(s).

Think of this pattern as a garden hose hooked up outside your house. When you turn the water on, it should flow freely through the hose. However, if you were to bend the hose, you would be creating a blockage. On one side of the bend, the water is blocked; on the other, there's no water at all.

This is what happens in your body if a blockage persists for long enough: It wears you out and depletes your Qi. For example, someone who is in a lot of pain is dealing with stagnation. Over time that person will become depleted and worn down both physically and emotionally.

Conrad came to my office seeking help for his chronic lack of energy. Some days he was so tired he just couldn't get out of bed. He came to me because he was worried about losing his job, having missed so much work due to his poor energy. He had several warnings from his employer about his attendance, and felt that getting fired was inevitable.

Conrad also struggled from depression and anxiety, and had done so for many years. He admitted to being irritable, restless, and a chronic worrier. Despite being exhausted, Conrad had a difficult time getting to sleep at night because his mind was full and his thoughts were racing.

Conrad also described feeling warm all the time, and would often wake during the night because he was hot and uncomfortable. All of his symptoms were worse when Conrad was stressed, which was becoming more frequent due to the possibility of losing his job.

When I began to treat Conrad, he regained some of his energy. However, a few weeks into treatment, Conrad was fired from his job. The stress and anxiety of being unemployed further aggravated his symptoms, making a complete recovery difficult at that particular time in Conrad's life.

Conrad's symptoms were due to a combination of Qi stagnation and Qi depletion. Symptoms pointing to his Qi stagnation included depression, irritability, and restlessness, which can cause a sensation of heat. However, the Qi stagnation was ultimately causing a severe Qi deficiency, as evidenced by his extreme fatigue and loss of energy.

If you are dealing with both stagnation and depletion, the best approach is to deal first with the stagnation, which is usually the underlying cause of your depletion. Some of the actions in this book may be helpful, but if the stagnation is longstanding, you may need to seek treatment from a Chinese medicine practitioner, who not only can offer acupuncture, but also can help with lifestyle and dietary changes.

CHINESE MEDICINE AND BLOOD

Another key substance that circulates in your body is Blood—both in Western and Chinese medicine. In both paradigms your Blood is responsible for nourishing and moisturizing every organ and all the tissues in your body.

The hallmark of Blood stagnation in Chinese medicine is pain that is fixed and stabbing in nature and is associated with blue or purple discoloration. A fairly benign example of stagnant Blood is a bruise. However, Blood stagnation can also affect your organ systems on a deeper level, as is the case with gynecological conditions or a heart attack. In the case of a heart attack, the fixed and stabbing pain is in the chest, and frequently a bluish discoloration is apparent on the sufferer's face and lips.

Treating Blood stagnation is a bit more difficult than treating Qi stagnation and usually involves acupuncture and/or herbal formulas. Frequently Blood stagnation is associated with more serious conditions, and I usually don't recommend self-treatment in those cases.

Blood deficiency is a condition in which your Blood is not adequately nourishing the tissues and organs of your body. In some ways, it is similar to anemia in Western medicine. Possible symptoms of Blood deficiency include a pale complexion, dizziness, insomnia, heart palpitations, numbness, dry skin, dry eyes, and brittle nails.

Blood can become depleted for a variety of reasons, especially in instances where Blood is lost, such as surgery, childbirth, heavy menstrual periods, or injury. In addition, chronic illness, poor diet, or poor digestion can deplete your Blood. Remember, it is through the digestion of nourishing foods that your body converts nutrients into Qi and Blood. If that digestive mechanism is impaired in any way, the long-term result will be depleted Qi and Blood.

A few years ago, Beth came to my office because she was experiencing heart palpitations several times during the day. These skipped heartbeats were alarming to Beth, even though her Western doctor told her they were nothing to worry about.

Beth was also having trouble with insomnia. She could fall asleep easily every night, but woke in the early hours of the morning and couldn't get back to sleep.

One year prior to her visit to my clinic, Beth had a hysterectomy for fibroid tumors. It had taken several months for Beth to recover her energy after the surgery. Since then, Beth noticed that her skin was much drier and her nails had become brittle.

Beth, a thin woman in her late forties, appeared extremely pale to me, and I could see that her skin was dry. When I asked about her diet, she told me that she ate healthfully and had been a vegetarian for over twenty years.

My diagnosis of Beth's imbalance was a Blood deficiency. She had lost a significant amount of blood during her surgery, and with a vegetarian diet, she most likely did not have the reserves to nourish and rebuild her Blood adequately. I worked with Beth for several months, combining acupuncture and herbs with some dietary modifications to nourish her Blood. During that time, her heart palpitations disappeared, and she was regularly sleeping through the night.

If you are suffering from Blood deficiency, your primary strategy is to nourish your Spleen system (See Chapter 6 on the Spleen) and to make sure you're eating and properly digesting nutritious foods. In general, dark fruits and vegetables, especially dark leafy greens, are nourishing to your Blood. Eggs and other high-quality (and low-fat) proteins such as black or kidney beans and lean meats are also good foods for nourishing Blood. Many foods that nourish your Yin (see Chapter 4) also have the ability to nourish your Blood. Blood deficiency is a condition that generally responds well to dietary therapy. Choose whole, colorful, and nutritious foods for the best results.

CHAPTER 4

BALANCING YIN AND YANG

You may have heard of Yin and Yang, or you may have seen the Yin/Yang symbol that looks like two fish, one black and one white, swimming together in a circle. Many people think that Yin and Yang arc just ways of describing opposites, but they're much more than that. Yin and Yang play a role in all aspects of your life, from your overall health, to how you age, how you sleep, and even how your skin looks.

To best understand the concept of Yin and Yang, consider the Chinese written character for each. Yang contains the elements of a hill or mound and the sun, indicating the sunny side of a hill. Yang, like the sunny side of the hill, is warm and bright. Because of the warmth, Yang moves upward and outward and is transforming. It's associated with activity, change, daytime, and the warmer, sunnier months of the year.

In contrast, the character for Yin contains the elements of a hill and the presence of clouds, which has been modernized and substituted with the element for the moon. Yin is represented by the shady side of the hill, which is darker and cool. The cool nature of Yin moves downward and inward, and is more nourishing. Yin is associated with rest or recovery, nighttime, and the cooler months of the year that have less daylight.

Yin and Yang are relative terms. For example, the new warmth of spring is considered Yang when compared to the cold, dark winter months. However, compared to summer, which is very Yang in nature due to its heat and longer, lighter days, spring is considered cooler and more Yin.

In your body, Yang is a force that is transforming and warming, a little bit like metabolism, and shares some of the properties of Qi. Yin, on the other hand, is cooling and nourishing and shares some of the characteristics of Blood. Body fluids are generally considered Yin substances due to their nourishing quality. You could say that the physical substances of your organs are relatively Yin, and the activities that your organs perform are relatively Yang.

The relationship between the Yin and Yang in your body is continually shifting. This relationship may be in good balance, indicating relatively good health, or it may become out of balance, causing you health problems and uncomfortable symptoms. As you age, the relationship tends to change, with Yin becoming depleted, leaving you to deal with the signs of a relative overabundance of Yang.

To determine if you have an imbalance between Yin and Yang, take the following quiz by checking off the items that are true for you.

Section 1

___I frequently have hot flashes or night sweats (waking up hot and sweaty).

___I tend to be constipated or to have dry, pellet-like stools.

___I often feel hot, especially in the late afternoon or evening.

___I often feel agitated and restless.

___I struggle with insomnia and feel restless at night.

___Often my mouth feels dry or I have a mild, dry sore throat.

___My hands, feet and chest feel hot.

___I have dry skin.

Section 2

___I am overweight by more than 30 pounds.

___I often feel colder than everyone else around me.

___I get up at night to urinate more than once, and my urine is clear and abundant.

___I feel like my metabolism is sluggish.

___My body frequently retains water.

___I have very little energy and feel sleepy all the time.

DEPLETED YIN, TOO MUCH YANG

If you checked one or more of the items in Section 1, it's likely that you have an imbalance with excessive

Yang in relation to Yin. Remember, a metaphor for Yin is the shady side of the hill. If you checked off any of the items indicating that you feel warm—whether it's warm hands and feet, having hot flashes, or waking up with night sweats—your Yin isn't cooling you properly and Yang is overheating. Yin acts like a coolant that keeps the Yang pilot light in check. When you have a shortage of Yin and a relative abundance of Yang, you will feel the effects as heat. Essentially, your radiator is starting to boil over.

Yin is quiet and contemplative, and Yang is active and moving. If you feel restless, are agitated, or frequently feel irritated, Yin is in short supply and Yang is acting up. Also, certain kinds of insomnia are related to having too much Yang. If you have difficulty falling asleep or staying asleep *and* feel restless and warm while you're trying to sleep, it is most likely related to Yang heat.

Yang as a source of heat can also cook the Yin fluids in your body, creating signs of dryness. A dry, sore throat, dry stools, and dry skin are all signs that your body has insufficient Yin. This is especially relevant to how you age, because Yin naturally decreases as you get older, and if you can minimize that decline, you'll feel and look better.

I frequently see women in my clinic who are in their early fifties and struggling with menopausal hot flashes and/or night sweats. This kind of heat is a classic example of too much Yang and insufficient Yin. As you get older, Yin naturally becomes depleted. However, during menopause, estrogen, which is a very Yin substance, drops fairly suddenly. This dramatic drop in cooling Yin causes a flare-up of Yang, which is warm and rising—exactly how most women would describe their hot flashes.

DEPLETED YANG, TOO MUCH YIN

If you checked one or more of the items in Section 2, your Yin may be overabundant in relation to Yang. Again, if Yang is your personal pilot light and Yin is a coolant, then when your pilot light is low it doesn't warm your body efficiently. Having too much Yin, or coolant, will actually make you feel cool. If you are always colder than everyone else or have to wear a sweater even on the warmest days of summer, your Yang may be depleted and not warming you very well.

Insufficient Yang is also associated with having too much water in your body. If your pilot light is low, you're not metabolizing fluids well, and this can show up in a couple of ways. You may retain water, such as swelling of your hands, ankles, face or under your eyes, or you may also find that you have to urinate a lot, even though you haven't had very much to drink. This may become apparent during the night

(Yin time of day) if you have to get up a couple of times to go to the bathroom, and you urinate far more than you have had to drink prior to going to bed.

Your body's inability to process fluids well can also show up as extra weight. Fat tissue is considered a Yin substance. If you are 20 to 30 pounds or more over your ideal weight, you are carrying a great deal of extra Yin and dampness around with you.

The warmth of Yang is responsible for the activity and movement of your body. If your Yang is seriously depleted, you may feel sluggish or chronically tired, or have the sensation of being unable to move.

Myra, a fit twenty-six-year-old woman, came to me because she was struggling with hypothyroidism, or a sluggish metabolism. Myra's primary concern was that she was gaining weight, even though her diet hadn't changed. In the past six months, she had gained about thirty pounds, and was very unhappy and puzzled by the sudden change in her health.

Myra also noticed that in the past several months she was incredibly tired all the time and constantly felt cold. She also noticed lately that her feet were swelling, especially after she had been driving for extended periods of time.

All of these changes were unsettling to Myra, because she considered herself a healthy and physically active young woman. Myra's Western doctor prescribed a thyroid medication, which seemed to slow her weight gain, but Myra still was not feeling like her old self.

Myra's pattern was one of deficient Yang. I treated her with acupuncture and heat on her lower abdomen, which helped to warm Yang and make her feel warmer overall. Over time, Myra's energy returned, and she began working with a personal trainer who helped her lose some of the weight she had gained.

WHAT YOU CAN DO TO BALANCE YIN AND YANG

To Nourish Yin

Besides acting to cool the body, Yin moves inward, nourishes, and soothes. Frequently Yin becomes depleted because you are not honoring those concepts. Becoming exhausted and overwhelmed can quickly deplete Yin, as can regularly becoming dehydrated or living in a very dry environment. In addition, Yin naturally declines as you age, so as you get older it becomes more important to do everything you can to nourish yourself.

The theme for anyone trying to rebuild Yin is to rest, rejuvenate and look inward. This means getting enough rest, sleeping seven to eight hours a night, and taking the time to nourish not only your body, but your mind and spirit. Yin's action is to move inward, and looking inward promotes Yin. Meditation, contemplation, grounding activities and quiet time are all great ways of promoting Yin.

If your Yin is depleted, you will want to eat foods that have a cooling and moistening effect on your body. Avoid coffee's stimulating effects, alcohol, and hot spices, all of which can be warming and drying. In general, choose colorful fruits and vegetables, which are nutrient-dense, moist, and nourishing, paired with small amounts of protein and carbohydrates. Some foods that nourish Yin and/or build fluids include:

Fruits
apples, apricots, Chinese wolfberries, lemons, mangoes, mulberries, oranges, pineapples, pomegranates, raspberries, pears, plums, strawberries, watermelon

Vegetables
alfalfa sprouts, artichokes, asparagus, avocados, peas, potatoes, string beans, tomatoes, yams

Grains
malt, barley, millet, wheat, spelt

Meat, Fish, and Dairy
cheese, milk, eggs, beef, duck, pork, rabbit, and organ foods such as kidney and liver, clams, crabmeat, mussels, oysters, sardines, scallops

Other Foods
black beans, kidney beans, seaweed, sesame seeds, sesame oil, coconut milk, soy milk, soybeans, tofu

For more information on balancing Yin and Yang through food, see *Recipes for Self-Healing* by Daverick Leggett and *The Tao of Healthy Eating* by Bob Flaws; publication information is included in the "Learning More" section at the end of this book. Both books are the source of the food choices listed in this and the following chapters.

A dish you might make to nourish Yin would be a congee, or rice porridge with a few drops of sesame oil, tofu, and mung beans paired with a fruit salad. Note: Go easy on the raw fruit if you have problems with digestion.

Basic Congee Recipe

Combine one part rice with seven parts water and cook over low heat until the rice is tender. For a complete meal, you can add broth and protein (chicken, tofu or egg), vegetables, sesame oil and herbs from the food lists to suit your taste and underlying imbalance.

Most herbs included here tend to be warming, especially ginger and scallions, so if you're trying to nourish Yin, use them in limited amounts or balance warm herbs with cooling vegetables. For example, you can offset the warming effects of ginger by adding mung bean sprouts to your congee.

For those of you who have problems with feeling too hot, here are some additional foods that have the action of clearing heat (Foods generally have more than one property. The foods that are on both lists both nourish Yin *and* clear heat):

Fruits
apples, bananas, grapefruit, lemons, oranges, watermelon (melons in general are cooling)

Vegetables
asparagus, bamboo shoots, cabbage, celery, cucumbers, eggplant, lettuce, mung bean sprouts, potatoes,

radishes, rhubarb, squash, spinach, tomatoes, water chestnuts

Grains
barley, millet, wheat

Meat, Fish, and Dairy
clams, crabmeat, yogurt

Other Foods
mung beans, marjoram, mint, peppermint, salt, soy sauce, tofu

Mung beans are especially cooling, so a soup made by cooking mung beans with some seasoned broth, barley, and potatoes would be perfect for clearing heat. Don't drain the water you used to cook the mung beans; just use it in the soup—it's very cooling.

The lists incorporated into this chapter are not the only foods with these actions. They were included because they are fairly common and can easily be included in your menu plan.

FOR DEPLETED YANG

Yang is warm and active, and it moves outward. In order to replenish Yang, you will need to warm, become active and move outward yourself. Activity is an important Yang concept, which may translate into physical exercise or moving your body in some way. Remember, movement creates heat, so find ways to get moving, whether it is stretching, walking in the woods or playing a game of tennis.

The concept of "active and outward" also may be interpreted as being motivated and out in the world. Your motivation for setting and achieving goals, your assertiveness, and how you approach challenges and obstacles are all fueled by Yang. If your tendency is toward quiet time and maintaining the status quo, it may be time to push yourself to take on some activities that feel risky.

One way to physically boost Yang is by stoking your pilot light. The source of both Yin and Yang in the body resides in the Kidneys, which are located in the small of your back. You can help strengthen the Yang in your body by applying heat to your lower back at about waist level. You can also apply heat to your lower abdomen about halfway between your navel and your pubic bone. Try to apply heat using a warm pack, rice bag, or hot water bottle twice a day (be careful to avoid burns!). I use heat in the form of an infrared heat lamp with my patients who feel cold, and their cold symptoms disappear fairly quickly.

You can also build up Yang by eating warm foods. Not only do foods have an inherent temperature, but the way they are prepared can exert a warming or cooling effect on your body. Raw foods are energetically cold. They take a lot of warming on the part of your body to be digested. In contrast, foods that are heated over a long period of time—for example, roasted foods—tend to be much warmer in nature. If you're trying to warm your body's Yang, try to eat more cooked foods, and avoid iced foods and drinks.

In general, eating proteins and whole-grain carbohydrates with smaller amounts of fruits and vegetables is best for replenishing Yang. The following is a list of some foods which have a warming effect on your body and help replenish Yang.

Vegetables
chestnuts, garlic, ginger, onions, scallions

Grains
quinoa

Meat and Fish
lamb, lobster, mutton, pheasant, shrimp, trout, venison

Other Foods
basil, chive seed, cinnamon, clove, cayenne, chili powder, dill seed, dried ginger, fenugreek seed, mustard, nutmeg, rosemary, sage, thyme, pistachios, walnuts

A great way to boost Yang is to combine some of these foods and spices in each meal. For example, lamb or mutton is extremely warming, so combining lamb and ginger in a stew would be a great (and delicious) way to warm Yang. Other combinations would be basil or chives sautéed with walnuts, or trout cooked with rosemary or sage.

In addition, if you have too much Yin, you may also have too much swelling, or edema. Some foods that have the action of draining water include:

Fruits
cranberries, grapes

Vegetables
alfalfa sprouts, broad beans, celery, lettuce, peas

Grains
barley, Job's tears (a grain similar to barley)

Meat and Fish
anchovy, clams, mackerel, sardines

Other Foods
aduki beans, black soybeans, kelp, seaweed, green tea, jasmine tea

A FINAL WORD

It is possible to suffer from a combination of depleted Yin and Yang at the same time. For example, you may retain water (a sign of Yang deficiency) *and* have night sweats (a sign of Yin deficiency). If you feel that this applies to you, consult with a practitioner of Chinese medicine, who will help you determine the best course of action, and how to treat your symptoms. Treating the greatest deficiency would usually be done first.

If you are suffering from a gross imbalance of Yin and Yang, in which the symptoms above are interfering with your daily activities, I would also recommend that you see a practitioner of Chinese medicine. Help can be offered in a number of ways, including acupuncture, which is highly effective for a variety of health conditions. Also, most practitioners are able to prescribe Chinese herbal formulas (be sure to ask) and can help you fine-tune your diet based on your individual symptoms.

CHAPTER 5
THE ORGAN SYSTEMS

OVERVIEW AND ASSESSMENT

Perhaps one of the most difficult concepts to explain in Chinese medicine is that of the organ systems. In our Western culture, when we talk about an organ, we tend to think of a physical entity that resides in a specific place in your body. In Chinese medicine, each organ has a physical place in the body, but it also has an energetic component, and the functions of an organ can be physical, emotional, or symbolic. Imbalances within an organ may manifest someplace in your body other than the physical site of that organ. An organ is first defined by the activities or functions associated with it, then by that organ's relationship with other organs, and last by its actual presence or location in your body.

Along with its physical functions, each organ has energetic characteristics that connect our bodies to nature in its own distinctive ways. Each organ is related to a specific element, such as fire, water, and the like, which gives the organ unique qualities. In addition, each organ is associated with a color, season, taste, sense, sound, and so on.

For the sake of simplicity, I have introduced only the Yin organs—the Spleen, Lung, Kidney, Liver, and Heart—which are responsible for the major processes in your body. Each Yin organ is paired with a hollow Yang organ—the Stomach, Large Intestine,

Bladder, Gallbladder, and Small Intestine. The Yang organs all have functions that are related to decomposing and moving food and waste through your body.

The energetic pathways which run along the surface of your body also run deep to connect with your internal organs. Therefore, when there is disharmony of one or more of your organs, they can be accessed through the pathways and acupuncture points on the surface of your body. Each organ has its own patterns of imbalance, some of which are excess in nature, such as stagnation, and some of which are depletion patterns. For example, patterns involving your Spleen are almost always ones of deficiency, and while your Liver can become deficient, it is more frequently an organ prone to stagnation.

To identify organ systems in your own body that may be out of balance and need some attention, take the following assessment by checking the statements that are true for you. The assessment will direct you to those organs that may need balancing and strategies for addressing some of the imbalances you uncover.

Check any of the statements that are true for you:

Section 1—The Spleen
___My energy is low.

___I tend to bruise easily.

___I frequently suffer from gas and bloating.

____I get tired after eating a meal.

____I seem to worry about everything.

____I have poor muscle tone or strength.

____I struggle with gaining, losing, or regulating my weight.

____My stools tend to be loose, or I have episodes of diarrhea.

____I don't have much of an appetite.

____My stomach rumbles a lot.

____Sometimes I feel sick to my stomach.

____My muscles feel weak.

____My digestion is poor.

Total for Section 1____

Section 2—The Lungs

____I have frequent sinus infections.

____I suffer from seasonal allergies.

____Other people tell me my voice is soft or weak.

____Grief is a common emotion that I experience.

____I seem to catch every cold or flu that's going around.

____I have asthma.

____I frequently feel sad.

____I sweat during the day, even when I'm not exercising.

____I frequently get bronchitis.

____I get short of breath doing simple tasks.

____I have a chronic cough.

____I can hear wheezing when I breathe.

Total for Section 2____

Section 3—The Kidneys

____I have a sore or stiff lower back.

____My ears ring.

____My hair is/has been thinning or falling out.

____I have been diagnosed with osteopenia or osteo-porosis.

____My knees are weak and/or sore.

____I feel afraid much of the time.

____My sex drive is low or nonexistent.

____I have or have had kidney stones.

____I experience frequent hot flashes or night sweats.

____I have hearing problems.

____I have been diagnosed with thyroid problems.

____Every night I get up several times to urinate.

____I have dark circles under my eyes.

____I feel cold all the time.

____I have infertility issues.

Total for Section 3____

Section 4—The Liver

____I frequently feel pain under or around my ribs.

____I sigh a lot.

____There is a bitter taste in my mouth.

____I tend to be inflexible in many situations.

____My eyes are dry, red, itchy or painful.

____I get migraine headaches.

____I am frequently irritable.

____I have been diagnosed with hepatitis.

____My joints and muscles are inflexible.

____(Women) Any symptoms I have are worse around my period.

____I struggle with depression.

____I have difficulty controlling my anger.

____My health problems are always aggravated by stress.

____I tend to have severe PMS.

Total for Section 4_____

Section 5—The Heart

____I have problems with my gums.

____Most of the time I feel hot.

____I experience heart palpitations, or the sensation of skipped heartbeats.

____My dreams are especially vivid or disturbing.

____I have pain in my chest.

____My urine tends to be pretty dark in color.

____I have had panic attacks or feel anxious.

____My entire face is red most of the time.

____My memory is poor.

____I struggle with insomnia most nights.

____I laugh or cry uncontrollably for no apparent reason.

____I can get confused or disoriented easily.

____I have sores in my mouth or on my tongue.

Total for Section 5_____

After you have completed the assessment, total up the number of items you checked for each section. The sections where you checked three or more items indicate organs that may have an imbalance, stagnation, or may need some building up. More checked items in a section are a stronger indication that you have an imbalance in that organ system.

Because the functions of your organs are so closely interrelated, it's not uncommon to have an imbalance in more than one organ system. If you checked several items in more than one section, it doesn't mean that your health is in peril; it just means that any imbalance you have is beginning to affect other organ systems.

The following chapters offer descriptions of each organ and its functions, symptoms of imbalances, and strategies to build up those organ systems that need your attention.

CHAPTER 6
THE SPLEEN

Think of your Spleen as the system that takes in nourishment and turns it into energy. It turns food and liquid into Qi and Blood. Your Spleen also receives emotional nourishment in the form of ideas and possibilities and turns them into opportunities and action.

Your Spleen accomplishes the process of digestion by sorting and separating, transforming, and nourishing. After its paired organ, your Stomach, has broken down what you have eaten, your Spleen separates the solids from liquids and the nutrients from waste. It then transforms the nutrients into Qi and Blood, which are sent on to the rest of your body. The strength of your energy and the nourishing quality of your Blood depend on the healthy functioning of your Spleen.

Another job of your Spleen is to hold things up, or hold things in place. It is your Spleen that keeps blood within the vessels, holds up organs, and keeps substances in their proper place. A weakening of this function might result in easy bruising, prolapsed organs (organs sinking downward), heavy menstrual periods, or chronic diarrhea.

Your Spleen nourishes your whole body, but it nourishes your muscles directly. If you have strong, flexible muscles with good tone, you can thank the health of your Spleen.

The sense associated with your Spleen is taste, which is the first step in the digestive process. As such, your tongue is the outward manifestation of the health of your digestion. The appearance of your tongue offers your practitioner of Chinese medicine a great deal of information not only about the state of your digestion, but also about your overall health.

Your Spleen corresponds to the element of Earth and the season of late summer. The Earth in the context of a farmer's field is the source of food that your Spleen digests, and harvest time, typically late summer, is the most nourishing time of the year. Your Spleen is also associated with the color yellow, which is the color of the Earth in many parts of China as well as the color of many of the nutritious fruits and vegetables that are harvested at the end of summer.

The emotional function of your Spleen is similar to the process of digestion. The emotional aspect of your Spleen is responsible for receiving and processing information, experiences and ideas. The ideas are "digested" or sorted and transformed into actions, intentions, plans, or goals. Other ideas are stored for later consideration, and the less useful ones are forgotten. Clear thought and acting with focus are signs that the emotional aspect of your Spleen is healthy.

When the process of sifting and sorting of ideas becomes overactive, worry is the result. Just like a cow in the pasture chewing its cud, worriers tend to ruminate over the same idea again and again. For some people excess worry has the potential to become anxiety, in which the sorting of ideas spins out of control, causing insomnia, fuzzy thinking, or even panic attacks.

Spleen pathology on the physical level is mostly related to poor digestion and its effects. Gas, bloating, rumbling, nausea, or the sensation of food not moving are all associated with a weak Spleen. Loose stools, diarrhea or in some cases constipation are also related to poor digestive function of the Spleen.

Fatigue is one of the results of a weak Spleen, as food transformed into Qi by your Spleen is the source of energy in your body. Feeling tired after eating, widely fluctuating energy levels, shortness of breath and poor energy in general can be indications that your Spleen isn't up to par.

If the transforming function becomes impaired, your Spleen may not metabolize liquids very well, and dampness may accumulate. In a farmer's field after a heavy rainstorm, the fallen rain should soak into the ground and nourish the crops. However, if the field is saturated, the rain will sit on the surface, make puddles and get boggy. In your body, the poor transformation of liquids creates dampness that can manifest as overall heaviness, fluid retention, diarrhea or loose stools, bladder or vaginal infections, and excessive weight gain.

While your Spleen is prone to dampness, its paired digestive organ, your Stomach, is prone to dryness and heat. When your Stomach heats up, it acts a little like an engine in overdrive. An insatiable appetite is the primary symptom of heat in your Stomach, but other symptoms of Stomach heat may include heartburn and sores in your mouth.

Brad, a busy salesman in his late fifties, came to my office looking for help for his digestive problems. He had struggled with stomach pains and diarrhea for years, and was willing to try anything—even acupuncture—if it would help his symptoms. Brad's appetite was poor, and whatever he ate seemed to just sit in his stomach. He frequently had stomachaches, bloating, and lots of rumbling.

Due to the nature of his work, Brad put in sixty- and sometimes seventy-hour workweeks, with a fair amount of traveling. He complained that when he was traveling, he was unable to eat healthfully because he was usually entertaining clients. As a result, many of his meals during the week were heavy and hard-to-digest foods paired with a number of cocktails.

He described his energy levels as good, but on further questioning, I found that Brad had just enough energy to get through the day. In the evenings, he was exhausted, and on the weekends, he took long naps to try to regain his energy.

Brad's pattern was one of Spleen Qi deficiency, most likely caused by overwork, poor diet, and travel. Brad's digestion improved over time with the help of acupuncture treatments, food therapy, and a plan for healthier eating when he was traveling.

NOURISHING YOUR SPLEEN

Because the Spleen is so closely related to digestion, food therapy can be especially effective in supporting its function. If you think of your Spleen as being related to harvest time and an abundance of food, then you will understand why comforting, satisfying foods are especially nourishing. Eating healthy foods you like in a relaxed atmosphere promotes good digestion. Also, food preparation can make a difference in your digestion. Soups, stews, and stir-fried meals are easily digested because they're well-cooked and don't overtax your Spleen's digestive function.

The color yellow is associated with the Spleen; its element is Earth; its season is fall; and the taste that's most nourishing to the Spleen is sweet. Knowing this, it makes sense that slightly sweet foods harvested in the fall from the Earth (root vegetables) that are yellow would be great food choices for people trying to improve the health and function of their Spleen. Good food choices include squash, carrots, potatoes, yams, turnips, pumpkins, and sweet potatoes.

While sweetness is the taste associated with the Spleen, it doesn't mean that the two-pound bag of M&M's or a big bowl of Cap'n Crunch is going to improve its functioning. Not so! To the ancient Chinese, sweet foods weren't measured in grams of sugar per serving, but were naturally sweet, like dates, carrots, squash, and fruits. While the sweet flavor is nourishing to your Spleen, eating too many sweets can actually damage it, causing dampness and overweight.

If you have a tendency toward dampness, avoid drinking too many fluids with your meals. By keeping foods and fluids separate, you are helping your Spleen in its sorting function. In addition, very cold foods and drinks are especially hard to digest. Your body has to use energy to heat up cold foods to a point where they can be digested, essentially sapping your body's energy in the process. Aim to eat and drink foods that are at least room temperature, especially if you struggle with digestive problems.

Finally, *how* you eat can play a role in supporting your Spleen. You should always eat sitting down and with good posture. Chew your food well to get the digestive process started. When you eat in a hurry, standing up and gulping your food, your Spleen has to work twice as hard to turn that food into nutrients.

Nourishing your Spleen emotionally involves connecting with the Earth. Feeling grounded, relating to nature, and centering activities all honor this element. The Earth element is also conceptually the center of the five elements. In this respect, feeling centered, attending to your home, and paying attention to structure and routines will nourish the Earth element. Pay attention to the routines in your life, clear out the clutter, and do small things to make your home or your space feel comfortable to you. Being away from home feels exciting at first, but ultimately, travel and homesickness can upset your Spleen.

I have had more than a few patients in my practice who struggle with being overweight *and* having clutter in their homes, seemingly unrelated issues. However, when they make the connection between the sifting and sorting function of the Spleen and how it affects not only their physical body but their surroundings, they are able to make progress on both fronts.

Getting outdoors and connecting with nature are activities that are also nourishing to your center. Take a walk, visit a local nature preserve, work in your garden, go camping, or choose any other activities that bring you into contact with the Earth element.

Your muscles also come under the realm of your Spleen. Strong, healthy muscles that are toned and flexible are signs of a healthy Spleen. Stretching, massage, and other forms of bodywork help to lengthen the muscles and open the flow of energy—and they feel really good, too.

According to Bob Flaws (*The Tao of Healthy Eating*, see "Learning More"), "Above all else, protect the Spleen." A healthy Spleen sets the foundation for abundant energy, strong Blood, and healthy functioning of all of the other organs.

CHAPTER 7
THE LUNGS

Of all the organs, the Lungs are considered to be the most directly connected to the exterior environment. Through the air you breathe, the outside world meets the inside of your body. When you get a cold or the flu, your Lungs are the first organ affected. Typical cold symptoms—a stuffy or runny nose, sore throat, and coughing or wheezing—are all related to your Lungs as they affect parts of your body through which air passes.

Your nose is the sensory organ associated with your Lungs. The acuity of your sense of smell is an indicator of Lung function. In addition, respiratory allergies or frequent sinus infections are also an indicator of the condition of your Lungs.

As the first organ affected by outside pathogens, your Lungs are also associated with your body's defense system, something called *Wei Qi* in Chinese medicine. Wei Qi is a bit like a protective bubble around the exterior of your body, working to fight off the germs that make you sick. If you tend to catch every cold that's going around, chances are that your Lung system and Wei Qi are not as strong as they could be.

As part of the exterior of your body, your Lungs are responsible for the health of your skin and hair (except that on your head) and for the opening and closing of your pores. If you tend to sweat easily or have problems with your skin, you may be having problems with your Lungs.

In Chinese medicine, the Lungs also regulate the water in the body. This may seem an unlikely idea, but if you put your mouth or nose up to a mirror, you'll see moisture on the mirror with each exhalation. Your Spleen separates liquid from the food you've eaten and transports it to your Lungs, from which location the liquid is gently precipitated throughout your body.

Even though water regulation is related to your Lungs, problems related to water retention may show up anywhere in your body. Dry, itchy skin, a dry mouth or dehydration in general are problems caused by too little water. Too much water can show up as swelling, edema, or phlegm. Phlegm is water that has been around for a while that has congealed, and while (believe it or not) phlegm can show up anywhere in your body, its most likely target is your Lungs. Asthma is a common condition affecting the Lungs, and in Chinese medicine it's considered a chronic phlegm problem.

The element associated with the Lungs is metal, and its color is white. Late fall is the season related to the Lungs. This is a time of change, or passing from summer to winter, much like the air passing through your Lungs with each respiration. Late fall is also a time of dryness. Because of the exterior positions of the organs associated with your Lungs—your nose and throat—these organs tend to become dry as well.

Emotionally, the Lungs are associated with grief or sadness. I have found in my own practice that when a patient is experiencing loss, it's beneficial to address the Lung system as part of their treatment.

Signs of Lung problems include coughing, wheezing, shortness of breath, sneezing, and chronic rhinitis or sinus infections. You can also consider the problem to be related to your Lungs if you have frequent colds or flu, asthma, bronchitis or a very weak voice. A weak physical exterior might show up as frequent or spontaneous sweating, and, in some cases, chronic hives.

Gerard, an eighteen-year-old high school senior and soccer player, came to me for help with his asthma, which made him extremely short of breath when he exercised. In appearance, he was a strong and healthy young man, but his voice was soft and it was often difficult to hear what he was saying. Gerard used an inhaler when needed, which helped with immediate symptoms, but his asthma didn't ever seem to get any better.

Gerard described himself as an easy sweater, and when I felt his pulse his skin was moist. Gerard also shared that he usually caught several colds during the course of the winter, and said that he frequently had bouts of unexplained hives.

Gerard's pattern was one of Lung Qi deficiency with underlying Phlegm. In all cases of asthma, there is an element of Phlegm. Gerard's symptoms were worse when he exercised, because he was further depleting his Lung energy. The Lung system also protects the exterior of the body, which was weak in Gerard's case, causing his sweating and chronic hives.

NOURISHING YOUR LUNGS

Perhaps the most obvious way to strengthen your Lungs is to use them. That's right, *breathe*. Whether through the intentional breathing of a Yoga class, singing, public speaking or exercising briskly, activities that open your diaphragm and cause you to breathe harder are good for your Lungs. While you're at these activities, open your chest and sit or stand up tall to enable your Lungs to pull in the air that is so vital to your well-being and to life itself.

Caring for your skin is also a way to nourish your Lung system. Brushing or scrubbing your skin to exfoliate and applying moisturizer daily are ways to keep your skin healthy.

As the organ that serves as the gate between the exterior and the interior of the body, the emotional aspect of the Lungs concerns boundaries. Feeling safe and being assertive are signs of healthy boundaries. So is the ability to say "no" when you want. Boundaries are also about respect—commanding respect from the people in your life, but also feeling respectful of others around you.

In some cases, poor emotional boundary issues can be the cause of certain kinds of illnesses. For example, chronic worriers are *over*reacting to perceived external threats. As a result, they may also overreact physically to perceived threats, making them prone to seasonal allergies, skin rashes and food sensitivities. People who *under*react to external threats may have difficulty asserting themselves. In the physical realm, this underreaction can translate into catching frequent colds and flu.

Grief, as the emotion associated with the Lungs, needs to be addressed. This may mean allowing yourself time to grieve after the loss of someone you love or the end of a relationship. If there's sadness in your life, acknowledging the cause, and spending some time with it—either through journaling or sharing your feelings with a trusted friend—are ways to come to terms.

Foods that are good for your Lungs are also foods that build up your Qi. Light proteins, such as fish or tofu, are helpful. White foods, such as white root vegetables, and mushrooms are also good for your Lungs. Pungent flavors are associated with the Lungs, so mildly spicy foods such as scallions, basil, ginger, and other strongly flavored herbs can be nourishing. If you tend toward dryness in your Lungs, fruits such as apples and pears are cool and moistening. In contrast, if you tend to have problems with phlegm, you'll want to avoid foods that engender phlegm. These kinds of foods include dairy foods, rich or greasy foods, and foods that have been overly processed.

Your Spleen is your connection to the Earth, but your Lungs are your connection to Heaven. Make time each day to consciously open your chest and breathe as a way to build your Qi.

CHAPTER 8
THE KIDNEYS

The Kidneys are the organ system of growth, maturation, sexuality, fertility, and aging. Like a seed which holds the potential of an entire plant, your Kidneys hold the genetic blueprint of who you are and how healthy and strong you will be.

Your Kidneys (or Kidney in Chinese medicine) are the source of Yin and Yang in your body. When the fire of Yang is burning low or Yin is not nourishing your body, your Kidney must always be addressed. Your Kidney also houses a substance called Essence, which is similar to DNA.

A Little Bit about Essence

Essence is one of the most important substances in the body, and is the foundation for all other substances—Qi, Blood, Yin, Yang, and Fluids. Essence is behind many of the functions of growth and development that are attributed to the Kidney, where it is stored.

You inherit one kind of Essence from your ancestors at the moment of conception, called Congenital Essence, which is responsible not only for growth and maturation, but also for genetic traits and constitution. When you work too hard, eat poorly, or become too stressed, and as you age, Congenital Essence becomes

---

depleted. When this Essence is completely used up, according to Chinese theory, you die. While Congenital Essence cannot be replenished, it can be used judiciously through good lifestyle habits, and it can be augmented by another kind of essence, called Acquired Essence.

Acquired Essence is made up of nutrients from the food you eat, and can be built up by eating well, getting adequate sleep, and acting with moderation in all things. Good health, strength, and high levels of energy are signs of an abundance of Acquired Essence. Any excess of Acquired Essence is also stored in your Kidney, along with Congenital Essence.

The Kidney is considered the most deep-seated of all the internal organs, and for good reason. It's the root of all substances in the body and is responsible for providing the tools you require to fulfill your deepest needs: survival and reproduction. Your Kidney acts a bit like the Energizer Bunny as the house of your deep reserves, but as such it's also the organ that is most damaged by stress.

Your Kidney is physically located in the lower back, so when it becomes weak, one of the most common symptoms is low back pain. Also, sore or weak knees or ankles can be associated with a Kidney weakness.

Your body's bones and marrow are governed by your Kidney. Weak bones and bone diseases such as osteoporosis are related to poor Kidney function. The function of your Kidney is connected to your ears and sense of hearing. When there is an imbalance or weakness in your Kidney system, a common symptom is tinnitus, or ringing in your ears. If you are losing your hair or it's going gray prematurely, you can also blame your Kidney, as it governs the hair on your head (not to be confused with your Lungs, which govern your skin and the hair on the rest of your body).

Your Kidney and Kidney Essence determine how well you will age. Gray hair, weak bones, loss of hearing, loss of skin elasticity, tooth problems, and many other signs of aging are related to your Kidney. If you are interested in aging as well as possible, your Kidney is the most important organ system to safeguard.

As the deepest, most interior of the organs, the color associated with your Kidney is black; its movement is inward; and its season is winter. The Kidney element is water, which is appropriate and symbolic in that water is the source of all life.

The organ paired with the Kidney is the Urinary Bladder, and together both organs govern water metabolism in the body. While the Lungs are assigned the task of water regulation, the balance between Yin and Yang is responsible for the actual metabolism of the body's fluids. If you think of Kidney Yang as a pilot light that warms your body and its fluids, then Yin is a bit like coolant, which nourishes your body and keeps the heat of Yang in check.

Sexuality and creativity are emotional components of the Kidney system. As the organ that governs survival through reproduction, the Kidney system is responsible for libido and sexual attraction. The Kidney is also the source of artistic creation. In addition, the emotions associated with this deepest organ are fear and fright. Fear has the ability to shake you to your core, and chronic fright translates into something very much like unrelenting stress, which is extremely damaging to your Kidney. In Western medicine, the adrenal glands pump out adrenaline and cortisol (stress hormones) and are located right next to the kidneys.

Signs and symptoms that your Kidney is depleted include a sore or weak low back, knees, or ankles; bone or tooth problems; dark circles under your eyes; hearing problems; and premature graying or thinning of your hair. Thyroid problems or extreme reactions to the climate—feeling really cold or having lots of hot flashes—are also indications that your Kidney is out of balance. Edema, kidney stones, and getting up several times each night to urinate suggest a problem with the water metabolism function of your Kidney and Urinary Bladder. Also, issues with fertility, libido, or your menstrual cycle generally are Kidney problems.

Sharon, a forty-two-year old woman, had a Kidney deficiency that caused a number of symptoms. When she was forty, Sharon, like Beth and many other women, had a hysterectomy for fibroid tumors. The surgery caused Sharon to go through menopause prematurely. Her sudden menopause, coupled with the recovery from surgery, depleted her Kidneys.

Sharon was a thin woman with an athletic build. She came to me because her knees hurt to the point where she couldn't exercise. Prior to her surgery and menopause, Sharon was an avid biker and runner, but the pain in her knees was making exercise difficult.

Almost as disturbing as her inability to exercise was the fact that Sharon's long blond hair was falling out and becoming extremely thin. In the past, she had gone through periods when her hair fell out, usually for a few weeks each fall. However, for the past several months, Sharon's hair was falling out by the handful, especially each morning when she showered.

Upon questioning, Sharon also said that she had mild hot flashes since her menopause, her ears were ringing, her lower back was achy in the early morning, and that she had to get up two or three times a night to urinate.

I treated Sharon's depletion of Kidney Qi and Essence with regular acupuncture, along with an herbal formula and food recommendations that nourish the Kidney. In addition, Sharon's very athletic lifestyle was contributing to her depletion, so I recommended that she change her exercise routine to include some less intense sessions of walking and Yoga classes.

During the course of several months, Sharon's knees felt better, and she reported that her hair loss had slowed considerably. Sharon also noticed that her hot flashes went away completely.

NOURISHING YOUR KIDNEY

Because your Kidney is the organ most damaged by stress, one of the best ways to nourish it is to get your stress under control. Whatever method you choose, whether it is Yoga, Tai Qi, meditation, or fishing, any stress relief measures will benefit your Kidney. Because it houses the source of Yin and Yang in your body, finding the right balance between activity and rest will help improve Kidney health. Yang activities include those that are challenging, exciting and stimulating; in contrast, Yin activities are those that incorporate rest, rejuvenation, and contemplation.

Beyond handling stress, dealing with any situations in your life that are making you fearful will only serve to enhance Kidney health. However, if you tend to be fearful with no obvious threat, trying activities that feel a little risky and stretch you beyond your comfort zone are also helpful.

The physical realm of your Kidney is your lower back and knees. Stretching and exercises to strengthen your lumbar area and leg muscles are helpful in supporting your Kidney. You can also stimulate your Kidney by patting or massaging your lower back area.

The color associated with the Kidney is black, and foods that are black or very dark are especially nourishing to this organ system. These would include dark fruits and vegetables, and foods like black beans, black sesame seeds and black walnuts. The water element comes into play when choosing foods for your Kidney. Foods from the sea, such as fish, shellfish, seaweed, kelp, and sushi are all excellent Kidney tonics. The flavor related to the Kidney is salty, which also speaks to foods from the ocean, but can also include other lightly salted foods and miso. Remember that some salt is helpful, but too much is damaging, and in this case, too much salt can upset the water metabolism function of your Kidney and result in high blood pressure. Foods that specifically nourish Yin and Yang are listed in Chapter 4.

Your Kidney is the organ system that most controls how well or quickly you will age, and the one action that can most affect its health is to manage stress.

CHAPTER 9
THE LIVER

The Liver is the organ system that governs the smooth movement of everything in the body. The first thing that comes into your head when you read "smooth movement" might be your bowels, which would be true. However, your Liver also governs the movement of digestion, the menstrual cycle and even your emotions.

In Chinese medicine, the Liver stores the Blood, which may seem like a strange concept, because you know that your blood moves throughout the body, and if it didn't, you would die. An easier way of thinking about your Liver's relationship to your Blood is that your Liver is responsible for the health and abundance of Blood. Essentially, if you have a deficiency of Blood (similar to anemia), it's usually a Liver Blood deficiency.

The Liver regulates the menstrual cycle (which makes perfect sense if you think of smooth movement and blood). Some of the key symptoms of Liver Qi stagnation for women are related to the menses. PMS, breast tenderness, irritability, and menstrual cramps are all symptoms that a woman may experience if her Liver energy isn't moving well.

The sensory organs associated with the Liver are the eyes. A strong, healthy Liver translates into good vision and healthy eyes. However, if you struggle with declining vision, dry, red or itchy eyes, cataracts, or other eye diseases, it would be important to explore your Liver system function.

The Liver harmonizes emotions, and emotional upsets are generally delegated to the realm of the Liver. Stress, while most damaging to the Kidney, is regulated by the soothing and smoothing qualities of the Liver. If you think of a time when you were under constant stress, chances are that you began to have physical symptoms, such as tight shoulders, neck pain, digestive problems, and irritability. These are all signs that your energy is stagnating and impacting your health.

The element associated with the Liver is wood, and for good reason. Like hard wood, the Liver is a strong organ system. Its function of smooth movement can be compared to the slow but steady growth of plants in the spring, or the slow but regulated rise of sap in trees. However, while appearing hard on the surface, wood must retain some flexibility or it will break, and this is also true of your Liver system. Without flexibility, whether physical or emotional, your Liver will stagnate.

Your Liver system controls the suppleness of your tendons and ligaments. Without the flexibility of your Liver, you may become prone to ligament injuries, pulls, and tendonitis.

The season associated with the Liver is spring and its color is green. The growing new shoots of plants that have been dormant throughout the winter are a good analogy for the action of the Liver system. It has the ability to move forward forcefully, but when hindered can stagnate easily and cause a wide range of symptoms.

Symptoms associated with the Liver include emotional issues, such as depression, irritability, and problems with anger. In addition, Liver symptoms are almost always aggravated by stress. Any problems that change or are worse around the menstrual cycle can also be attributed to your Liver. Eye problems are Liver issues, and if you get migraine headaches, chances are that they're related to your Liver, too. The Gallbladder is the organ paired with the Liver, and can produce symptoms like constant sighing, pain under your ribs, and a bitter taste in your mouth. Shingles and hepatitis are considered Liver/Gallbladder problems that have combined with dampness and heat.

The emotional landscape of the Liver is strong and assertive. However, when the strong and assertive nature of the Liver is thwarted, depression or anger may result. Most people who struggle with depression have some degree of Liver stagnation.

The nature of the Liver is to move forward force-fully, and it is human nature to want to move forward throughout life unimpeded. However, the greatest source of emotional stagnation is the inability to move forward. Your Liver drives your self-realization, and when there is a great divide between how you think things should be and how things really are, the opportunity for your Liver to stagnate is very real. When your potential or sense of purpose is obstructed, the result is anger. The key to damage control is flexibility. If you are able to yield to the realities of your life, to plan to move forward, but to revise that plan when necessary, then you will be able to move through life smoothly.

Jennifer came to my clinic several years ago for help with depression; she wanted to stop the antidepres-sant medication she had been taking for several years. She felt that while the medications helped with her depression, their side effects upset her digestion.

Jennifer was a bright and outgoing woman in her mid-forties. She worked at a stressful job in which she frequently felt powerless, and her husband was a frequently unemployed computer technician. Jen-nifer shared with me that she was struggling in her marriage, and was generally unhappy with all aspects of her life, but felt unwilling or unable to make any changes.

Beyond depression, Jennifer's symptoms included a constant pain around her ribcage, a bitter taste in her mouth, and poor digestion. Jennifer ate healthfully most of the time, but she had chronic diarrhea that seemed unrelated to the foods she had eaten. She exercised regularly and tried to meditate daily. All of Jennifer's symptoms were worse when she was under stress. In fact, Jennifer concluded that her symptoms were probably the direct result of the stress in her life.

The difference between the way Jennifer wanted her life to be and how it actually was created a pattern of Stagnation of Liver energy. Jennifer's symptoms were improved greatly with acupuncture and Chinese herbs. She was able to go off of the antidepressant medications for several months at a time until some stressful or upsetting event occurred. In the long run, because her circumstances remained unchanged, Jennifer's underlying pattern of Liver stagnation did not completely resolve.

NOURISHING THE LIVER

The secret to Liver health is flexibility. This includes both flexibility in your thinking and physical flexibility. Emotional flexibility might be expressed through creative endeavors and through trying to see things from another viewpoint. Physical flexibility can be accomplished through stretching and specific disciplines like Yoga, Pilates, Qi Gong, and Tai Qi that work to lengthen your muscles and strengthen your tendons and ligaments.

If you're prone to stress, which is the hallmark of Liver stagnation, movement is the obvious remedy. Emotional movement, or flexibility, can provide a different way of thinking about what's stressing you, or inspire a different way of coping. Physical movement is especially helpful when you feel things stagnating. Almost everyone who exercises feels physically and mentally better afterward. That's because moving your body is moving your body's energy. You do not have to become a marathoner to have exercise work for you; taking a walk, working in the garden, or paddling a canoe all qualify as energy-moving activities.

Foods that nourish your Liver are those that have the ability to cleanse. Sour foods (the taste associated with the Liver) help your Liver release toxins and stimulate your Gallbladder to excrete bile, which is used in breaking down fats in your diet.

Green is the color related to the Liver, and spring is its season, so eating new plants that have sprouted early in the spring are especially nourishing to your Liver. Sprouts, salads, greens, and early plants are Liver foods. Also, because the health of the Liver is associated with the health of the Blood, foods that nourish Blood are beneficial. In combination with Spleen-nourishing foods, dark fruits and vegetables, leafy greens, meat, eggs, legumes, and whole grains are all beneficial in nourishing your Blood.

Combining diet with flexibility, stress management, and movement are the keys to keeping your Liver energy moving smoothly.

CHAPTER 10
THE HEART

From a purely medical standpoint, we usually think of the Heart as an organ that pumps blood and is prone to heart attacks as we get older. In Chinese medicine, however, the Heart is the organ system that houses the *Shen*, which is the mind, memory, consciousness, and spirit. While these activities are attributed to the brain in Western medicine, we tend to intuitively know that the Heart is also an organ of feeling or spirituality. In fact much of our language about the Heart refers to it as an organ of feeling. Terms such as someone "tugging on our heartstrings," "knowing things in your heart" or having a "broken heart" are speaking to an emotional organ rather than simply a muscle that pumps blood. Of course, the Heart does move Blood throughout the body, but that function is secondary to its job of housing the *Shen*.

The health of your Heart is reflected in your face. It is said that you can look into someone's eyes to see the spirit, or Shen, of that person. The sensory organ related to the Heart is the tongue. Your Spleen is assigned the sense of taste, but your Heart's relationship with your tongue is in its ability to form words—a way of projecting your Shen.

The element associated with the Heart is Fire, and as such it is a warm and active organ. Its activity is responsible for moving Blood throughout your body, but it is also the activity of your mind and the warmth of your body which animate you as a human being. The color related to the Heart is red (an obvious choice) and its season is summer.

The emotion associated with the Heart is joy, which can be a double-edged sword, in that too much joy can become mania. As the home of your Shen, your Heart is your connection to your spirituality, your connection with the universe, and your relationship to the divine, however you choose to define it.

Because the Heart is the home of consciousness, it has some relationship to most emotional disturbances, notably anxiety and insomnia. When you become out of touch with reality to the point of mental illness, your Heart is always involved. When you are unable to connect with reality, it is considered a "misting" of your Heart, a term for loss of clear thinking and cognizance.

Pathology associated with the Heart includes palpitations, insomnia, vivid dreams, chest pain, and gum problems. Heart pathology may also reflect the Fire element, including signs of excess heat in your body, such as feeling hot, thirst, dark urine, craving cold foods and drinks, and a red face.

Carrie came to my office a few years ago because she had a habit of laughing inappropriately and being unable to stop. At the beginning of Carrie's first appointment, she seemed joyous and happy, but after about twenty minutes, it became apparent that she was unable to calm down and stop laughing. In fact, the harder she tried to control her laughter, the worse it became.

Carrie was in the process of looking for jobs in her field and was worried that she wouldn't be able to stop laughing during job interviews. She shared that the more overwhelmed she felt, the worse the laughter became, but that she could control this to some degree by thinking peaceful thoughts. She had an important interview coming up the following week, and was trying acupuncture as a last resort.

Carrie was in her twenties and very healthy, but she had been in a traumatic car accident about six months before coming to me. She had healed from her physical injuries after the accident, but she was still troubled by the traumatic nature of what had happened. Carrie said that after the accident, she had become very jumpy and the laughter had begun.

During her first appointment, I learned from Carrie that she felt hot most of the time and was very thirsty for ice-cold drinks. She had difficulty getting to sleep and once she was asleep, she would wake during the night hot and sweaty.

I diagnosed Carrie with a Heart pattern, because her *Shen*, or spirit, had been greatly disturbed by the accident. After three or four appointments, in which I treated Carrie with acupuncture, she was much calmer and able to control her laughter almost completely. She was able to successfully interview for positions in her field, and had some job opportunities that she was considering.

NOURISHING YOUR HEART

The key to nourishing your Heart is in connection. Connecting with your sense of purpose through journaling and self-exploration, connecting with others in social situations, and connecting to the divine through prayer and meditation are all nourishing to your Heart. Celebrating the seasons and spending time in nature are also ways of connecting with creation. Finding ways in your day to be joyous is honoring your Heart and the Shen within.

Nutritionally, foods that bring joy feed your Heart. Meals that have been prepared with love, foods you love to eat, and gathering with friends and family for a meal are all Heart nourishing. The taste associated with your Heart is bitter, the taste of that which has been burned. Bitter foods such as especially dark chocolate and bitter greens are stimulating to your Heart. Red foods and beverages derived from red foods are also good for your Heart, so stock up on tomatoes, red peppers, apples, a little (very little) red meat and red wine.

The next time you are full of joy or feel something with all your heart, remember that in Chinese medicine, your Heart is actually the keeper of all your feelings.

CHAPTER 11

TONGUE AND PULSE DIAGNOSIS

Part of making an accurate diagnosis in Chinese medicine involves your practitioner looking at your tongue and feeling your pulse. Both tongue and pulse diagnoses can offer information about the state of your health. Usually, the conditions of your tongue and pulse serve to confirm a diagnosis that your practitioner has already made. However, in some instances, your tongue or pulse may offer additional details that help your practitioner make a more complete diagnosis.

For example, Erik came to my office several years ago for pain relief from a shoulder injury. His shoulder pain had been a nagging nuisance for the better part of a year, but had recently gotten much worse. Erik had a job in which he traveled almost every week, and his shoulder pain was making it hard for him to lift his luggage.

At his first treatment, when I finished talking to Erik about his shoulder and his overall health, I had a fairly clear idea as to how I would treat him with acupuncture—that is, until I asked to see his tongue. Erik's tongue was red with a thick and patchy yellow coating, which was not at all what I expected to see. The red color and thick coating told me there was more going on with Erik's health than just a shoulder injury. The appearance of Erik's tongue indicated that he had dampness and heat in his body, most likely due to poor digestion. In Erik's case, the dampness and heat could cause or aggravate the pain in his shoulder. This caused me to go back and ask more questions and revise my treatment plan for him.

Many of my patients have asked me what I see after looking at their tongue or what I've found after feeling their pulse. This chapter serves only as an explanation of those processes, and should not be used to diagnose or treat yourself or others.

TONGUE DIAGNOSIS

During your first acupuncture treatment, your practitioner will usually ask you to stick out your tongue. While this may seem like an odd request, the color, shape, and coating of your tongue provide a great deal of information to your practitioner.

The appearance of your tongue is fairly accurate in reflecting the condition of your interior organs and digestion. In addition, changes in the appearance of your tongue can indicate improvement or deterioration of your particular imbalance.

Certain areas on your tongue loosely correspond to your internal organs, with the tip of your tongue reflecting the health of your uppermost organs. The condition of your Heart is determined by looking at the extreme tip (or point) of your tongue. The area corresponding to your Lungs is also at the tip, but behind the very point of the tongue. The very center of your tongue corresponds to the center of your body, your Spleen; and the back of your tongue reflects the health of your Kidneys. Both sides of your tongue indicate the health of your Liver.

A normal tongue is pale red and fresh-looking. It should look supple when it's extended. It should not quiver, have deep cracks, or be too flabby or thin. A normal tongue coating is white and thin, and may be slightly thicker at the back of the tongue. A normal tongue will also appear moist, but not too wet.

Some signs that your practitioner will consider when looking at your tongue include:

Color

The color of the body of your tongue is probably the most accurate indicator of the true state of your health, especially when your practitioner is presented with conflicting symptoms. In general, a red tongue indicates heat somewhere in your body. An extremely red or crimson tongue means that the heat is severe. In contrast, a pale tongue can be an indication of deficient Qi and/or Blood, or an indication of a cold condition. A tongue that appears purple or bluish is a sign that there is a stagnation, or impaired flow of Qi and/or Blood.

Form

The form, or shape, of your tongue body is often a clue to the state of fluid balance in your body as a whole. A tongue that appears enlarged, fat, swollen, or scalloped on the sides indicates edema, or dampness. If the body of your tongue is small and/or thin *and* red, then fluids are depleted. This usually means a Yin deficiency combined with heat. A small, pale tongue is an indication of energy (Qi) or Blood deficiency. Fissures or cracks in your tongue also indicate a deficiency of fluids, especially if your tongue also appears dry.

Bearing

The bearing of your tongue when it is extended is also an important clue to the status of your overall health. While infrequently seen in the clinic, a tongue that appears stiff, limp, or hard to control can be an indication of neurological issues. This is also true of a tongue that deviates to one side when it's extended—which is frequently seen in a patient who has experienced a stroke. In Chinese medicine, this kind of tongue would indicate interior wind.

A trembling or quivering tongue that is very red can be an indication of Yang moving upward and causing internal wind. However, a trembling tongue that is pale usually indicates an energy deficiency.

Coating

Both the color and the texture of your tongue coating offer numerous clues as to the internal condition of your health, especially the quality of your digestion. It is important to remember, however, that the color of your tongue or its coating can be affected by foods like orange juice, coffee, red wine, and, more obviously, by food dyes (especially bright blue or emerald green!). If you are looking at your tongue, be sure to note if you have eaten anything that may artificially affect the color of your tongue or its coat.

A white, clean, moist and thin tongue coating is considered normal. If your coating appears yellow or brownish, then heat has cooked the coating and indicates the presence of some kind of heat in your body, possibly Stomach heat. A black tongue coating is rare, but usually indicates a severe condition, and must be evaluated with other signs and symptoms.

A wet, shiny tongue coating is an indicator of moisture in your body, either dampness, phlegm, or not enough Yang to cook fluids. In contrast, a tongue coating that appears dry can be pointing to either internal dryness or heat.

In general, very thick tongue coatings indicate stronger pathogenic processes at work in your body. A tongue coating that is very thick and slimy usually indicates strong phlegm or dampness. It also points to a problem with your digestion and the transformative processes within your body.

A tongue that has no coating or appears shiny and peeled is a good indicator that heat has damaged Yin or fluids.

Combining Tongue Signs

In making any kind of tongue diagnosis, a complete picture must be taken into account. For example, a pale tongue with a thick and greasy-looking coating may indicate phlegm combined with cold, or food stagnating. However, a thick and greasy coating on a red and swollen tongue would more likely indicate damp and heat or phlegm and heat.

It's also important to look at where on your tongue the coating is the thickest, where it is peeled, or where cracks are appearing. For example, a deep crack in the center of your tongue points to heat in your Stomach, but cracks on the sides of the tongue may be Liver fire.

Tongue color may not always be evenly distributed. For example, a pale red tongue with a very red tip (frequently seen in the clinic) indicates a disturbance in the Heart—often related to anxiety or an emotional upset.

Changes

Changes in the appearance of your tongue are helpful in determining the status of your health. In general, tongue appearance is slow to change when dealing with internal conditions or imbalances of your organs. However, with an external illness, like a cold or the flu, the appearance of your tongue may change more rapidly. For example, someone with the flu who is running a fever may have a very red tongue until the fever subsides. In contrast, a patient who is being treated for internal heat may find it takes longer for the red appearance of their tongue to change.

I had been treating Jeff, a regular patient, for about a year. Recently he came to me for a severe muscle pull in his hip. He had pulled the muscle playing tennis about three weeks before; the injury was so severe he could barely walk.

In his late forties, Jeff was usually very healthy. He ate well and was physically active most days. He was sick infrequently, and used acupuncture as a way to stay well. His tongue was usually light red with a thin white coat.

During Jeff's third treatment for the muscle pull, he became extremely short of breath. He shared that he had experienced a similar episode the previous evening, in which he felt pain in his rib cage and short-ness of breath. I immediately stopped the treatment and urged Jeff to get emergency medical care, which he did.

The emergency doctor diagnosed Jeff as having an injury or muscle pull between his ribs, and pre-scribed a pain medication. The doctor also informed Jeff that an injury of this type would take several weeks to heal.

Jeff continued to see me during this time. He didn't like taking the pain medication, because it upset his stomach and made it burn. In addition, Jeff complained that he just didn't feel right, and rather than getting better over time, he was actually feeling worse.

During this period, I examined Jeff's tongue on several occasions. His normally healthy tongue had taken on a bluish hue and had a vivid red spot right in the center. As time went on and Jeff didn't improve, his tongue became a dark bluish-purple in color, and the red spot remained. This change in Jeff's tongue was somewhat puzzling; his muscle pull was a stagnation that could cause his tongue to take on a bluish or purple color, but Jeff's tongue had become *really* dark.

After several weeks, Jeff had had enough of not feel-ing well, and with my urging, he went to his regular doctor for a full physical. His doctor ordered a number of tests and sent Jeff to a lung specialist. The lung specialist diagnosed the pain in Jeff's chest as a blood clot, probably from the deep muscle pull in his hip, which had traveled to one of his lungs, causing the lung to fill with fluid—a potentially life-threatening condition.

With this diagnosis, the change in appearance of Jeff's tongue now made complete sense. His normally light-red tongue had become blue and eventually dark purple, because he had a major stagnation in his chest, which was impeding his ability to breathe. The red spot in the center indicated the irritation to Jeff's Stomach caused by the pain medications he had been taking.

Jeff ultimately made a complete recovery, not only from the blood clot, but also from the muscle pull in his hip. The bluish-purple appearance of his tongue changed back to pale red over time, and the bright red spot in the center faded as his Stomach recovered.

PULSE DIAGNOSIS

The quality of your pulse can offer your practitioner of Chinese medicine a great deal of information about the strength of your energy. Taking a pulse is complicated, as there are almost thirty different kinds of pulses—many of which are difficult to distinguish from one another.

On the positive side, pulse diagnosis can be more exact than tongue diagnosis, because the different positions of the pulse indicate the status of specific organs. The most frequent site for pulse diagnosis in Chinese medicine is the radial pulse on the underside of your wrist. A practitioner will always use three fingers to feel your pulse, keeping the middle finger even with the knob of your radial bone. The index and ring fingers will fall naturally into the two positions on either side of the middle finger. Your wrist pulse is divided into three positions, which correspond to the following organs:

Left	Right
Heart	Lung
Liver	Spleen
Kidney Yin	Kidney Yang

Note: These positions begin behind the crease at your wrist and move back the width of a finger tip towards the direction of your elbow. Your Heart and Lung positions are closest to the crease of your wrist.

Detected differences in pulse quality between the various positions give your practitioner a clue to the status of your underlying organs. For example, if your pulse feels strong in every position except the one closest to the wrist crease on your right, your practitioner might suspect a weakness in your Lungs.

Describing all of the types of pulses is beyond the scope of this book, but the following sections will give you a general idea of what your practitioner is registering when taking your pulse.

Rate

When you go to your Western medical doctor's office and the nurse takes your pulse, the purpose is to measure the beats per minute, or pulse rate. This is also the case in Chinese medicine, but your pulse rate is usually measured in relation to your rate of breathing. In general, a normal pulse rate is four to five beats per breath (inhalation and exhalation). A pulse that is markedly faster frequently indicates heat or an excess of Yang Qi somewhere in your body. A pulse that is slower usually indicates a cold condition, a deficiency of Yang, or possibly too much of a Yin pathogen, such as phlegm or dampness.

There are several factors that can naturally affect the rate of your pulse. Athletes, for example, tend to have much slower pulses than the general population, and this is not considered an imbalance. Also, small women can have a slightly faster pulse, which is also not a problem.

Depth

Have you ever tried to feel someone's pulse and had a hard time finding it? It is likely that you had trouble because the person had a deep pulse. The level at which your pulse is felt can offer some important clues to the location and nature of an imbalance. A pulse that is only felt deeply—meaning you have to apply pressure to find or feel it—indicates that an imbalance or disease is in the interior, and the organs are probably affected.

When your pulse is easily felt without applying any pressure, and it is not felt if more pressure is applied, then your pulse is considered to be floating. This indicates that any pattern affecting your body is very exterior in nature—such as a cold or the flu. The next time someone you know gets the flu, ask to feel his or her pulse; it will likely be floating.

Force

The force of your pulse indicates the nature of your energy, or Qi. A pulse that feels weak or forceless is a common indicator of a Qi or Blood deficiency. A soggy pulse is one which is felt easily but feels spread out and soft. It is also an indicator of Qi or Blood deficiency, or, in many cases, dampness. An extremely thin or fine pulse also points to a deficiency, which can be of Qi, Blood, Yin, or Yin and Yang together.

In contrast, a full, lively pulse that is easily felt indicates a healthy abundance of energy. It's possible, however, to have too much of a good thing. A pulse that feels wiry or extremely tight, like a guitar string, is common in someone who is experiencing severe pain or someone with a Liver pattern—usually stagnation—which indicates a lot of stress or an emotional upset.

Putting it Together

As with everything else in Chinese medicine, it is the combination of factors that reveals the most information. Your practitioner will take into account the rate, depth, quality, and differences among the various positions in reaching any conclusions from your pulse diagnosis. For example, a pulse that is rapid, deep, thin, and barely felt in the left rear position could be interpreted as a deficiency of Kidney Yin with some heat (remember, Yin is cooling). The rapid rate indicates heat, the thin quality points to a deficiency, the depth suggests an imbalance of the interior, and the lack of pulse in the left rear position narrows the deficiency down to the Yin aspect of the Kidney.

I had been seeing Greta, a lively woman in her late fifties, for over two years. Greta had been suffering from chronic headaches for over forty years, and acupuncture really helped decrease the frequency with which these headaches occurred.

One day Greta came into my office complaining of feeling really hot—hotter than her regular hot flashes. When these periods of heat subsided, Greta said, she felt chilled. In addition, she reported feeling dizzy over the past couple of days.

I was puzzled about these new symptoms: Were they just a different manifestation of the Yin deficiency and heat from which she suffered, or was this something else? Feeling Greta's pulse gave me the answer. Usually her pulse was somewhat tight and deep—felt only with a little pressure. However, today Greta's pulse was right on the surface, and when I applied pressure, the pulse disappeared.

Greta had what is called a floating pulse. Her pulse, combined with the feverishness and chills she described, indicated that Greta was fighting off an exterior pathogen—some kind of virus or flu. Greta's pulse gave me the information I needed to make a clear diagnosis.

Chinese pulse diagnosis is a subtle art; it takes years of experience for a practitioner to become proficient. There are infinite pulse variations, which can make interpreting the nuances of your pulse very difficult. For more detailed information about pulse diagnosis, I recommend *The Web That Has No Weaver* by Ted Kaptchuk (see "Learning More").

CHAPTER 12
PUTTING IT ALL
TOGETHER

At this point you may be thinking, *Okay, I know about Yin and Yang, Qi, and the organs, but how does an acupuncturist figure out where to stick the needles?* The answer is that it's a process in which the outcome is based on countless variables. Let's start with a diagnosis.

The first order of business in Chinese medicine is determining exactly what is out of balance. Imbalances are described as patterns, or a constellation of signs or symptoms describing your particular disharmony. It is possible to have more than one pattern at a time, and frequently one pattern will be the cause of another.

A practitioner of Chinese medicine will arrive at a diagnosis through a detailed interview in which you'll be asked questions about your primary symptoms as well as your physical and emotional health. You might be asked about your energy levels, how you sleep, your appetite and digestion, and your mood. At the same time, your practitioner is looking for visible signs that indicate a pattern—is your face red or pale, are you agitated, is your skin dry, and are your eyes dull or bright? Information will also be collected by listening to the quality of your voice and the clarity of your lungs. If your breath or body has any distinctive smells, that will be noted as well.

Your practitioner most likely will examine your tongue for clues about what's going on inside your body. Your practitioner will also feel the pulses on your wrists in order to gather information about the strength and quality of your energy. Your pulse might feel very taut and firm or very deep and hard to find—all indicators of the state of your health.

In diagnosing a pattern, a practitioner must consider a number of variables. One common method of diagnosis is called the Eight Principle Pattern Diagnosis, which really is a series of four dichotomies:

- **Is the pattern one of excess or deficiency?** Is there too much of a pathogen or substance, or is there not enough? For example, stagnation of Qi is considered an excess pattern because it has created a blockage, and Yin deficiency is an obvious lack of the substance of Yin.

- **Is the pattern internal or external?** Colds and flu are considered external patterns, because your body is trying to fight off a pathogen that has invaded from the outside. Internal patterns are generally related to your organs and substances such as Qi, Blood, Yin and Yang. Your pulse can be a good indicator here—a pulse that feels like it's floating on the surface usually indicates an exterior pattern, and a deeply felt pulse indicates an internal imbalance.

- **Is there heat or cold in this pattern?** Although some imbalances are neutral in temperature, many have a hot or cold quality. Examples of conditions that create warm patterns might be inflammation or fever, and cold illnesses might be accompanied by chills or a feeling of deep cold.

- **Is it a Yin pattern or a Yang pattern?** A Yin disharmony would have more Yin qualities such as dampness, cold, edema, or phlegm, indicating too much cold and moisture. A Yang disharmony would have too much heat and dryness—fever, inflammation, thirst, and irritability—more Yang characteristics.

Your practitioner will be able to determine your pattern based on each of these four sets of variables. For example, you may have a deficiency of Qi, which is a deficiency pattern, is internal, cool (as Qi is slightly warming) and is a mild Yin pattern, again because the warming quality of Qi is lacking.

A Note about Pathogens

As stated earlier, pathogens are a little like bad weather in your body. They can come from outside (like a cold or flu) or from the inside, and can make you sick.

The common pathogens are:

Heat: Heat can take the form of inflammation, infection, fever, and restlessness. Some signs that heat may be present include a thirst for cold drinks, irritability, and a rapid pulse.

Cold: The opposite of heat, cold is usually manifested as feeling cold, but can also produce certain pain conditions, sluggish metabolism, and a slow pulse.

Dryness: Often the result of heat or a prolonged illness, dryness indicates a lack of fluids in your body. Manifestations include thirst, dry mouth, dry skin, and an unproductive cough.

Dampness: The result of poor water metabolism in your body, dampness is like a field that doesn't drain well after a rainfall and pools in different parts of your body. It can be difficult to resolve. Symptoms of dampness include a lack of thirst, a heavy feeling, edema, yeast infections, and in some instances diarrhea or loose stools.

Phlegm: Often caused by dampness congealing, phlegm can be visible or invisible. Visible phlegm collects in your lungs after a cold, but invisible phlegm can cause a host of symptoms from nausea to lumps and even mental problems.

Summerheat: A pathogen that's unique to the warm weather, summerheat can manifest in a couple of ways. One form is caused by exposure to intense heat in the summer, and its symptoms are very similar to those of heat stroke. The other form comes from a combination of hot weather and humidity, with symptoms such as fatigue, nausea, and dizziness combined with symptoms of dampness.

Wind: This is a pathogen having many characteristics of the wind, but manifesting in your body. The onset of wind is usually sudden with rapid changes; it comes and goes, and usually affects the upper part of your body. Some of the symptoms of wind include tremors, shaking, dizziness, itching, "wandering" pain, and numbness. External wind is also a player whenever you have a cold or the flu.

On another level, your practitioner must determine if there is any organ involvement in your diagnosis. Each organ has been discussed in previous chapters, and each has hallmark symptoms indicating an imbalance. For example, a hallmark symptom of Heart involvement is palpitations, and a hallmark symptom of a Kidney imbalance is weakness or pain in the lower back or knees.

Adding organ systems into the mix narrows the diagnosis further. You might have a Kidney Yin deficiency, which is deficient, internal, warm, and a Yang pattern of your Kidney. This pattern is warm and more Yang, because the cooling qualities of Yin are depleted.

Another consideration for the practitioner of Chinese medicine is which pathways are involved. This is especially important if you have a pain condition, in which your pathways are obstructed.

The system as it's described here may sound fairly straightforward, but in reality it can be quite complicated for several reasons. First, most people have a combination of patterns—it is rare in the clinic to see a patient who clearly exhibits only one pattern of disharmony. Second, most imbalances, if left untreated, cause other imbalances. Third, imbalances change, and once you begin treatment, that change may be accelerated.

CHOOSING ACUPUNCTURE POINTS

Acupuncture points are like "on and off ramps" to your body's energy pathways. By needling into various points, your practitioner can access both your pathways and deeper organs. Which points to needle are determined by a number of variables such as the following:

- Local or distant points: Generally, a mix of points is used, some near the area of pain or imbalance and some farther away on your body.

- Pathways involved: If a pain condition is being treated, then pathways affected by the pain might be chosen. For conditions involving your organs, various pathways might be used. Many pathways go deep and connect with your internal organs, and almost always points on more than one pathway will be chosen.

- Function of each point: Each acupuncture point has specific indications or actions. Points with a desired action will be chosen based on your particular pattern.

- Combinations of points: Many acupuncture points work in combination with others. Again, a pair or set of points might be used for their ability to enhance a treatment when combined.

- Preference of the practitioner: Acupuncturists often use the particular points which work best for them in the clinic. This relationship between the acupuncturist and the points chosen is an important aspect of each treatment.

- Style of acupuncture practiced: The style of acupuncture your practitioner uses will also determine which points will be chosen. For example, Auricular acupuncture uses points located in your ear, Korean Hand acupuncture is limited to your hand, and practitioners of five-phase acupuncture tend to use only points below your elbow and knees.

THE TREATMENT

Once your practitioner has arrived at a diagnosis, treatment can begin. After selecting the acupuncture points to be used, your practitioner will insert the needles, which will be retained for twenty to thirty minutes—sometimes more. The needles are sterile, and most states require that they be disposable—used only once and then discarded (rather than sterilized and used again). The needles used for acupuncture are very thin in diameter, about the breadth of a thick strand of hair. Some people are concerned that acupuncture will hurt, but most people who have had acupuncture would not describe it as painful. The needles may cause some sensation while being inserted, but in many cases they are not felt at all. While receiving treatment, you might feel a dull or thick sensation at an acupuncture point as your body's energy connects with the needle. Most patients find acupuncture extremely relaxing, and some people even fall asleep during their treatment.

Depending on your condition and the style of your practitioner, you may be prescribed an herbal formula or some other additional therapy, such as dietary counseling, heat, bodywork or cupping. Cupping, as mentioned earlier, is a method of moving stagnation by applying glass or plastic cups in which suction has been created. The most common area to cup is the back, but cups can also be applied to other areas of the body.

Most people want to know how many treatments they will need to resolve their health condition, and this can be a hard question to answer. Because acupuncture is stimulating your body to heal itself, how quickly you respond to treatment is very individual, and is generally based on how healthy you are in the first place. Also, acute conditions—those that have been a problem for only a short time—tend to resolve faster than a condition that you have had for several years. Combining therapies such as acupuncture and herbal medicine tends to speed the healing process, too. Usually you will know after a few treatments whether acupuncture is helping your condition.

FINDING THE RIGHT ACUPUNCTURIST

You may be reading this book because you have had acupuncture and you want to know a little more. Or you may be thinking about trying some alternative treatments for a health condition and exploring how acupuncture and Chinese medicine work. For most people, Chinese medicine may feel risky because they do not know much about it, and finding a practitioner might feel a little like gambling. Choosing an acupuncturist can be overwhelming, especially if you have never had acupuncture before. It is important to ask some questions before you book an appointment for an acupuncture treatment to make sure you are getting the right practitioner for you and your particular needs. The following are some questions to ask a prospective practitioner before you book your first appointment.

- **What are your education and licensure in acupuncture?**

  This is an important first question to ask anyone who might perform acupuncture on you. All too frequently consumers are led to believe that any practitioner who is trained or certified to practice acupuncture is highly qualified in the arts of diagnosis and treatment using the principles of Chinese medicine. Do not hesitate to ask prospective practitioners about their credentials and training.

Physicians are required to have only100 to 200 hours of training in the technical use of acupuncture prior to using it as a treatment. This is considered "medical acupuncture."

Many chiropractors advertise that they offer acupuncture. It is important to know, however, that depending on which state you live in, they may be required to have only 100 to 150 hours of unspecified training in acupuncture. They typically take a test sponsored by their local chiropractic board to become certified. Chiropractors who perform acupuncture call themselves "board certified acupuncturists." In addition, they are usually legally limited to performing only acupuncture treatments that augment chiropractic adjustments.

Licensed acupuncturists (LAc) are required to have a minimum of 1,800 to 2,400 hours of education and clinical training, depending on the state of their licensure. They must also be board certified with the National Certification Commission for Acupuncture and Oriental Medicine (NCCAOM), a national regulatory agency governing Oriental medical education and credentials, and they are licensed by their state's Board of Medical Practice.

Licensed acupuncturists practice internal medicine, which focuses on the underlying source of your problem rather than just treating symptoms. As a result, they can treat a variety of conditions beyond the simple pain relief offered by most chiropractors and medical acupuncturists.

Most licensed acupuncturists must also have a master's degree in either acupuncture or Oriental medicine. The distinction between the two is that a practitioner with a master's in acupuncture is trained primarily in acupuncture. A practitioner with a master's in Oriental medicine is trained both in acupuncture and in diagnosis and treatment using traditional Chinese herbs.

- **Do you have a specialty? What are your experience and success with my particular condition?**

Some acupuncturists treat any and all conditions. However, many specialize in treating certain conditions, such as muscle and joint pain, stress and anxiety, infertility, or women's conditions. It is important to ask whether a prospective practitioner has had some experience treating your condition.

- **What kind of acupuncture do you practice?**

Most people don't know that there are many different kinds of acupuncture, such as traditional Chinese acupuncture, ear acupuncture, Japanese style, Korean Hand acupuncture, cosmetic acupuncture, and scalp acupuncture. Some of these disciplines are more effective than others for specific conditions. For example, Ear acupuncture is especially successful in treating addictions, such as quitting smoking and losing weight, and scalp acupuncture might be more valuable for conditions affecting the nervous system. Be sure to ask which conditions are best helped by your practitioner's kind of acupuncture.

- **How many treatments will I need?**

No practitioner should answer this question on the phone before seeing you, taking your health history, and making a diagnosis. In fact, everyone heals at a different pace. Your condition may be resolved in one or two treatments, or it may take many more, especially if it is a long-term, chronic condition.

- **Do you accept insurance?**

Many health care plans currently don't pay for acupuncture treatments. As a result, many acupuncturists are fee-for-service providers. If you think your health insurance plan may cover acupuncture, check to be sure. Make sure the acupuncturist you ultimately choose will accept your insurance as payment or provide you with a receipt so you can be reimbursed by your health plan.

If you have a health savings plan, acupuncture qualifies for reimbursement. Be sure to ask your acupuncturist for a receipt.

CHAPTER 13
SIMPLE STEPS

The attempt to distill the concepts of Chinese medicine into clear, simple ideas and descriptions of actions has expanded my appreciation of its complexities. My intention in writing this book is to give readers a basic understanding of Chinese medicine and some simple ways to use the practices of this medicine to become healthier.

The very nature of Chinese medicine makes this tricky, because one of the basic concepts is that everyone is unique. Each of us comes with our own body constitution, strengths, weaknesses, and tendencies. As a result, any recommendations made here come with the caveat that above all else, you must pay attention to your presenting pattern and/or underlying tendencies. For example, if you've experienced damage to your Kidney from working long hours under stressful circumstances, then improving your digestion will not be enough to bring you back into balance.

I recommend that after reading this book, you seek out a practitioner of Chinese medicine/acupuncture and get a clear diagnosis or description of any imbalances you're experiencing. If you're struggling with uncomfortable symptoms or a health condition, this is especially important.

The Simple Steps to better health include the following:

- Take actions to treat your specific imbalance. Again, this may require the help of a licensed acupuncturist or Chinese herbalist; seeking out a qualified practitioner would be well worth the effort to make sure you are on the right track.

- Support the function of your Spleen. This means taking the necessary actions to improve or protect your digestion. Energy in the form of Qi and nourishment from the Blood are made primarily from the foods you eat. Choosing the right foods for you and cooking them in ways that are easily digested are crucial in promoting good health.

- Soothe your emotions. The Chinese say that the emotions are the cause of 100 diseases, and for good reason. Strong negative emotions such as anger, fear, frustration, anxiety, and even stress can cause your energy to stagnate and make you sick. From treating patients in my clinic, I could safely say that stress alone is the source of more than 100 diseases. Take the steps necessary to alleviate the situations that are distressing you.

- Keep everything in moderation. Remember, a little sugar nourishes your Spleen, but too much chocolate cake can be damaging. In the same vein, the right amount of exercise is a bit like the fountain of youth, but exercise in excess can be extremely depleting. Too much of anything can be damaging over time—aim for variety.

- Change the behaviors that are making you sick. This may be more difficult than it sounds, because you have to determine what is making you sick, and then you have to make the commitment to change. I frequently see patients who know that their stressful lifestyle and long work hours are the sources of their poor health, but who are unwilling or unable to change. However, if you fail to remove the cause of an imbalance, symptoms of the imbalance will continue to surface.

- Balance the Yin and Yang in your life. This translates into getting enough physical activity and mental stimulation during the day, as well as getting enough sleep at night. It also means being out in the world, taking risks, and trying new things, while at the same time finding ways to look inward, meditate, visualize, and nourish your soul.

- Finally, pay attention to the natural world around you. This is the foundation on which Chinese medicine is built. Pay attention to the seasons and their corresponding elements. For example, in the fall eat foods from the Earth that are local and have just been harvested, especially yellow foods such as squash, carrots, and sweet potatoes. In the spring, celebrate the active and expanding energy of Wood by getting outdoors for your favorite physical activity. At the same time, keep in mind that extreme weather has the potential to create imbalances. For example, Summer-heat occurs during the hottest (and usually most humid) days of the summer, and damp conditions are aggravated during damp and rainy weather. Remember, the natural world is reflected in your body.

LEARNING MORE

The following books serve as my bibliography and are also great resources for further reading. Enjoy!

Flaws, Bob. *The Tao of Healthy Eating.* Boulder, CO: Blue Poppy Press, 1998. Bob Flaws explains Chinese dietary therapy in a clear way that's easy to implement.

Kaptchuk, Ted. *The Web that Has No Weaver: Understanding Chinese Medicine.* Lincolnwood, IL: Contemporary Publishing Group, 2000. This book offers an excellent detailed explanation of Traditional Chinese Medicine. I frequently refer to the section on pulse diagnoses, as it's the best I've seen.

Leggett, Daverick. *Recipes for Self-Healing.* Devon, England: Totnes Press, 2004. This is a great source of specific foods for each individual pattern and includes easy and delicious recipes.

Liu, Jilin and Peck, Gordon, Eds. *Chinese Dietary Therapy.* Edinburgh: Churchill Livingstone, 1995. A little more detailed than Flaws's book, *Chinese Dietary Therapy* includes very specific actions for most foods.

Maciocia, Giovanni. *Tongue Diagnosis in Chinese Medicine, Rev. Ed.* Seattle, WA: Eastland Press, 1995. This is a great resource if you are looking for more information on Chinese Tongue Diagnosis, and it includes photos.

ABOUT THE AUTHOR

Professionally, Lynn Jaffee has promoted good health for over two decades. She is a nationally certified and state licensed acupuncturist and Chinese herbalist in addition to being certified in the Mei Zen method of cosmetic acupuncture. She received a master's degree of oriental medicine from the Minnesota College of Acupuncture and Oriental Medicine in Bloomington, Minnesota. As a public speaker, Lynn has presented to groups of all sizes on topics related to acupuncture and Chinese medicine. Widely published in trade publications and periodicals, she is the co-author of *The Bodywise Woman*. She has an acupuncture practice in St. Louis Park, Minnesota and is married with two sons. They live in Hopkins, Minnesota.

Made in the USA
Charleston, SC
27 January 2012